LOOK THE DEMON
IN
THE EYE

LOOK THE DEMON IN THE EYE

The Challenge of Mid-Life

ANGELA NEUSTATTER

Illustrations by Christine Roche

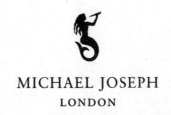

MICHAEL JOSEPH
LONDON

MICHAEL JOSEPH LTD

Published by the Penguin Group
27 Wrights Lane, London w8 5TZ
Viking Penguin Inc., 375 Hudson Street, New York, New York 10014, USA
Penguin Books Australia Ltd, Ringwood, Victoria, Australia
Penguin Books Canada Ltd, 10 Alcorn Avenue, Toronto, Ontario, Canada M4V 3B2
Penguin Books (NZ) Ltd, 182–190 Wairau Road, Auckland 10, New Zealand

Penguin Books Ltd, Registered Offices: Harmondsworth, Middlesex, England

First published in Great Britain 1996
1 3 5 7 9 10 8 6 4 2

The author and publishers wish to thank Faber & Faber Ltd for permission to reprint extracts
from 'East Coker', 'Burnt Norton' and 'The Love Song of J. Alfred Prufrock' by T. S. Eliot from
Collected Poems 1909–1962

Typeset in 11/13.5pt Monophoto Sabon
Typeset by Datix International Limited, Bungay, Suffolk
Printed in England by Clays Ltd, St Ives plc

A CIP catalogue record for this book is available from the British Library

ISBN 0 7181 3760 4

The moral right of the author has been asserted

For Olly with love, for sharing (he says suffering), the turbulent, unpredictable and often enriching mid-life journey with me. And for our sons, Zek and Cato, who have no idea what this ageing business is all about but think we are definitely over the hill.

Contents

Acknowledgements

Heartfelt thanks go first to Cate Kelly, who helped me far beyond the usual scope of a researcher with her tremendous diligence and energy, her intelligent thoughts and comments and her remarkable equanimity when I asked the unreasonable of her. Thanks too to the other researchers who helped at different times: Sophie Hastings; Andy Nurse; Namita Chakrabarty; Alison Chapman; Hannah Renier; Ashe Hussam; and Cos Michael.

I am very appreciative of the time and effort Hilary Mackaskell put into reading the manuscript and making perceptive comments. I have also valued greatly the kindness of close friends who have offered time to read bits, their thoughts and voices, encouragement and – well – friendship and I hope they will recognize themselves in this description and feel duly appreciated.

I owe much gratitude to the Centre for Policy on Ageing, Age Concern and Leonie Kelleher, editor of *Generations Review*, for their willing help as well as the information and documents they have let me have. Henry Fenwick, editor of *Modern Maturity* in Los Angeles, was kind and cheering when we met during my researches there.

Woman's Journal and the *Guardian* generously allowed me to place requests for people to make contact with me as subjects for the book and others responded to my advertisement in *The Oldie*. I am, of course, hugely indebted to the very many people who so kindly wrote me letters, filled in my hideously cumbersome questionnaire and invited me into their homes, or visited me in mine, to answer all manner of impertinent questions. Their words, thoughts, philosophies and experiences are the rich meat of my book.

Christine Roche has brought her perceptive and witty view of things to this book with her illustrations for the chapter headings, and I am more than grateful for this added dimension.

And, of course, thanks to Louise Haines and Rory Smith, my editors at Michael Joseph, both of whom have been a delight to work with, but who, I suspect, have aged considerably through working with me on this project. Thanks too to Jane Bradish-Ellames, my agent at Curtis Brown, who has been ever available and valuable to call on at tricky times.

Introduction

It never occurred to me that I would become middle-aged. It wasn't in the scheme of things for us, the post-war bulge and baby-boom generations who had grown up with youth as the Gold Standard and the belief that we had the Peter Pan quality. Mid-life, if we thought about it at all, seemed remote – it was what happened to the older generation. But the inevitable has happened; biological time has chuntered on, and a sizeable percentage of all Europeans and of Americans are mid-lifers. And that includes me.

So, now that it has come upon us, what do we think about it? How are we dealing with it? Does it have any significance as a life-stage? And can we, generations who have pioneered so many changes in our lives, make mid-life – which has tended to be seen as the scrag-end of youth, the beginning of fade-down time, defined only by the hiccup of a possible mid-life crisis – into something constructive?

We are unique generations, and there are many reasons why we will experience mid-life quite differently from previous generations. We have had more education, greater opportunities, better health; and, with the expectation of greater longevity, mid-life is likely to be a substantial chunk of our lives, extending beyond the forties–sixties, which, thus far, have generally been agreed to be the middle decades. We are also the generations who have been active and vociferous about asserting the right to be who and what we are.

Time magazine, in a feature on the new mid-lifers, referred to us as the Command Generation, seeing a confidence and competence, a sense of ourselves, which are the outcome of the way we lived our earlier years; certainly, for a good many people, this is a part of the picture.

And yet, far from feeling in command, many of us find ourselves feeling chronologically dispossessed, too old to be called young any longer, too young to be called old. It feels like an important time, but it is afforded no importance. And what those optimistic purveyors of good cheer about mid-life fail to grasp is that, no matter what rewards we may have garnered from the years of living and experience we have had, ultimately at mid-life we must come to terms with the fact that, inevitably, we will become elders and must then face our own mortality.

And for our generations, for which youth was made to seem the only thing worth having, the fear of the demon ageing that we face at mid-life is probably greater than it has ever been: the pain we may experience in grappling with this, and in finding a way of coming to terms with it in one way or another, is explored in the two chapters 'Critical Time' and 'Look the Demon in the Eye'.

I believe that mid-life can and should be an important era in our lives, and this book is intended to look at how we may make it that. As I see it, we have a choice between ignoring mid-life, and hoping it doesn't really exist, and embracing it, turning it into a particularly valuable time of assessment and preparation.

On the one hand, it is, in developmental terms, a critical life-stage, and we can take on board the psychological lessons we encounter and prepare ourselves psychologically and spiritually for a new time that requires new approaches. And, on the other hand, we can use mid-life in a very practical way, as a time for planning and designing how we want the next stage of life to be, from becoming political about the way older people are treated to framing ideas for ways of living that are alternatives to isolation and loneliness. Finally, I have drawn together the thoroughly upbeat, inspiring evidence I have found that later life may be an altogether more stimulating, fascinating and enjoyable place than I ever thought in my youthful days.

I see this as a book about choosing how we may re-order our lives and find new opportunities – though I am all too aware of how limited such choices are for the far too many people who have to live with crippling poverty, debilitating ill health and stresses that blight their lives. Although this was a personal exploration, it seemed to me essential, if it was to say anything of value to others, that it must include a breadth of feelings, thoughts, experiences. With this in mind, I interviewed more than 150 people of different types, classes and creeds. It is true that many came from my own circle, which would be classified as white middle-class. But the views of people from ethnic minorities and from less privileged classes are represented.

At the end of it all I now find myself going through mid-life and feeling better about it, and about the prospect of going forward on my journey, than I did when I began. This book has led me to find some useful tools for growing older, while making the trajectory. I hope it may do the same for others.

NOTE: The names of some people interviewed have been changed as requested.

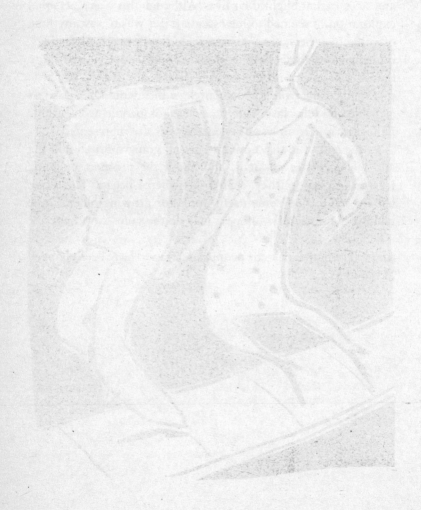

Too Long in the Tooth for Nirvana

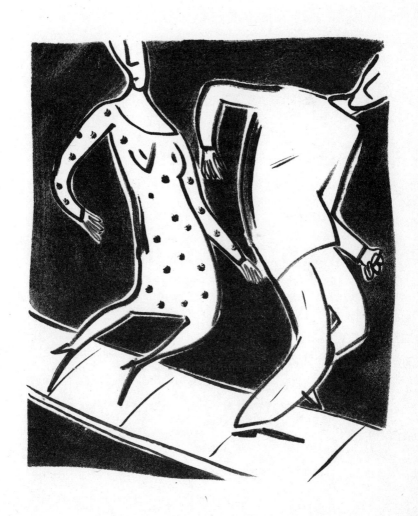

I caught sight of myself in the mirror the other day, not
realizing for a moment it was me, and I thought who's that old
bugger? Outrageous! That can't be me. I'm only twenty-five inside.
HUGH WHITEMORE, PLAYWRIGHT

I CELEBRATED MY FORTIETH birthday in high spirits and
a clingy, glitzy outfit. No way did I mind being forty.
Stepping over the mid-life Rubicon might worry other people,
but it wasn't my problem – that was the sartorial and verbal
statement, loud and clear. And I convinced myself.

But it was not so simple. Within a couple of years my
equilibrium seemed to have gone AWOL, my certainties
appeared to be on shifting sands. I felt a profound, but
incomprehensible discontent with all that I had striven for
and worked to build up, even though nothing, apparently,
had changed.

It did not occur to me at the time that this might have
anything to do with the fact I had hit middle age and, whether
I liked it or not, was embarked on an important developmental
journey at the end of which I would be an elder. But as I began
to discuss how I felt with my peers – men and women and
some from quite different backgrounds from my own – I
found I had company. Women opened the floodgates on their
fears as to who and what they would be in a few years, what
the empty nest might mean. Those who had chosen not to
have children and had felt sure-footed in this decision throughout their twenties and thirties, those who had not been able to
have them whether for physical reasons or for lack of a
suitable partner at the appropriate time, were wondering what
a future without this family link would mean. Mid-life had
been the catalyst for some unmarried women to experience
their first real anxiety about a future being single – and single

3

men similarly found this. But other people on their own believed they found mid-life less worrying than some couples with children, who were faced with having to find a new way of shaping life once that phase ended. Some questioned whether they could find a way to an emotional fulfilment which seemed to be lacking. But as often as people focused on a particular issue as the reason for discordant feelings, there were many like me, bemused in the face of their seemingly illogical discontent.

My kids' former childminder, who had always struck me as a person whose well-organized, sociable, family-oriented life would provide all the support she needed into old age, suddenly confessed a raging discontent and yearnings she dared not openly admit to. Most unnerving of all, she said, she found many of the mothers of the children she had cared for, her contemporaries, going through precisely the same.

The fear of being signed off from experiences that had stirred emotions in a way we wanted to go on experiencing, concerned many of us, and were articulated for me over dinner in a New York restaurant, where an elegant, composed woman executive I scarcely knew leaned across the table and confided: 'The thing I yearn for most is passion. I just want to experience those feelings which you felt confident would come by again, sometime, when you were young. If I see a film in which there is tremendous sexual and romantic intensity I can be in pain for days just longing to have those feelings again.'

We laughed wryly about this accepting, *tant pis*, that it is how things are. Later, through the many interviews I carried out with women who had passed through mid-life, I began to see the feelings my New York acquaintance longed for just might still be an option for women, and men, as they age. My interviewees laughed in quite a different way when I related this story to them – their laughter was at us for our foolishness – and told me of love affairs conjuring precisely the same feelings they had had when younger.

The men were no less eager to talk about what mid-life

meant to them, but they were inclined to speak with greater distance describing feelings of being disconnected, bleak, as though their feelings were blanked out much of the time, and they seemed fearful of acknowledging yearnings or uncertainties although some did. Their anxieties were often related to the business of achievement and the tussle within themselves if they did not feel they had matched their own expectations. For some it was quite unbearable to recognize that they had not achieved as much as others. Duncan Meadows, a secondary school teacher, pitched into despair soon after his fortieth birthday, and it was then that he began questioning the value of who he is: 'I ask myself whether I have achieved as well as I might have done, whether I have been a good enough parent, have I developed relationships of the depth I could have done? I have had this very powerful feeling that everyone else was going somewhere and I wasn't.'

Gordon Liss, who runs a small business and is in his late forties, surveys a long-standing marriage, teenage children he talks of with great pride, a pleasant home and says bleakly: 'I feel as though I am wrapped in grey membrane, suffocating, and I don't see what will change that unless I change my life. But why should I want to do that? It makes no sense.'

Over and over the mid-lifers talking to me echoed my own sense of puzzlement at what was going on, even though their ways of expressing it may have been different. Not everyone, of course, feels this way as they move into the fifth decade when mid-life is generally seen to begin. It is defined by those evaluating life stages as between forty and sixty. But of course nothing is absolutely clearly defined and there is a considerable number of people who describe their critical times as taking place in their fifties, while others believe they have come to it in their late thirties.

Psychoanalyst Peter Hildebrand conducted a workshop on the problems of the second half of life at the Tavistock Clinic, London, over nearly twenty years. He has seen that there are issues around ageing with which many people feel the need of help, support and the possibility of sharing and exploring what is going on in order to face the future and live it constructively. He has found as I have that if we take courage and face the fact that we are ageing and explore the issues around it, we can not only look forward to a future as an elder which will be rewarding and enriching, but that we can continue to grow and develop. He takes fifty to seventy-five as his period for growth which is logical, given that it is now suggested that the increased longevity we expect will push what we define as mid-life forward. 'What is needed is greater public recognition of the emerging problems of the years between fifty and seventy-five, which the French have christened the Third Age. Human beings in our time are enjoying and living through a period for which there are no precedents and we have to begin to deepen our understanding of the psychological variables which are involved. He believes we can look forward to a period of time in the First World when it should be possible for the ageing population in the Third Age to demand and acheive a leisure-based period of creativity and service which will be far longer and more productive than any similar group has achieved.'

But we do not so easily look forward from the perspective of mid-life, for we have not yet cut ourselves free from the investment and involvement we have with our younger years, nor from our yearnings to hold on to these. Hildebrand states that: 'Ageing is an intricate, delicate and on-going process, in which we and others constantly interact with and confront our solutions from the past, our prejudices from the present and the pressures from the inside and outside.' The onset of that ageing process is mid-life, I maintain, and throughout the following chapters I set out to show why the issues which arise at mid-life, while not necessarily exclusive to this period, have a particular meaning because of the point we are at in our life-cycle. My aim is to explore the idea of mid-life as a time of emotional and physical transition, a time when we must negotiate a significant change of status from that half of life lived as a younger to the second part during which we move on to become an elder.

There are people for whom the transition is, apparently, something which happens as a seamless follow-on from the younger years. When I have discussed my findings and beliefs these people have tended to look at me askance, or to brush aside the idea that mid-life is per se problematic and perhaps suggest that the whole idea of mid-life angst and upheaval is the psychological posturing of over-indulgent generations.

One may be glad that they feel this way and recognize that their feelings mean mid-life does not have to cause emotional turmoil, but I do not accept the dismissive view. There is too much serious long-term work on the human condition that discusses the middle-years as having a particular developmental significance, for me to accept that I have manufactured a syndrome to suit my purposes.

Added to this my own research convinces me that what has been described over and over in terms of a profound distur- bance of the soul is considerably more significant than mere posturing.

There is too little research into mid-life as such for us to gauge much about how generations before have felt, but there are good reasons why we, the West's bulge-and-boom genera- tions, the never-had-it-so-good kids, the post-war pioneers who cut our teeth on agitprop politics and helped create a culture to suit our youthful selves should find mid-life and middle-age difficult to come to terms with. We have grown up believing we were THE generation that counted, that centre stage was our sinecure for life and that somehow eternal youth, or at least protection from the experience of being less valued than the generations who inherited the youth mantle, was to be our legacy. But mid-life has arrived for us and although there are distinct signs that we are changing the rules, and that we probably feel more feisty, up-and-at-'em, and confident than generations before have been, we are nevertheless having to recognize that we are ageing.

The irony is that, having been the generations who helped create and colluded in the propagation of youth supremacy, we have sown the seeds of our own painful mid-life destruction. Bryan Appleyard, writing in the *Independent*, expressed the dilemma neatly:

In the post-war years, being young has become not simply a phase but rather the central experience in life. The discovery of the economic power of the young in the 1950s and 1960s led to a systematic glorification of the adolescent experience in films, television and music. The social and sexual intensity of those years was celebrated as the core of the modern self, the high point of contemporary experience . . . Youth culture became absolutely separate, deliberately disconnected from the rest of society. The end of youth became the end of everything.

With such a value system it was hardly surprising that ageism set in, and it is we, the bulge-and-boom generations, who are experiencing its real impact. The deification of age has led to the denigration of age, and that is one powerful reason, I believe, why mid-life is difficult to accept and why we can see little to welcome in the idea of maturing into later life.

Add to that the fact that across Europe and America, as we erstwhile youth generations targeted and feted because of our economic power, move towards senescence, we are being told in no uncertain terms that we represent a potential large-scale problem for the future. Where the generations before us growing old, post-Beveridge's reforms, have been able to believe in a future in which they would be provided for, as we age we hear what a problem our future welfare represents. Almost daily some politician or other is talking about how impossible it will be to provide for the unpleasantly named grey explosion.

On top of all this it is at mid-life that many of us really face mortality for the first time. It is the time when, commonly, people see parents dying or friends who are not so far from their own age. We become aware of the things that can go wrong with the body, the illnesses that may be terminal. People have talked to me repeatedly of this being the time they face their own mortality. Whereas, as young adults, we see death as something that happens to other people, at mid-life it is something that will happen to us.

We may not consciously worry about these things but I am convinced that reaching mid-life and recognizing that these are issues that we must confront, along with the psychological transition which must be made, are some of the reasons why today's mid-lifers may find it a harder time than generations before have done.

I am not suggesting that with mid-life we step into an era of unmitigated gloom and doom, an enclosed dark tunnel of the human spirit. Indeed there are for many of us times when the very fact of maturity may feel like an achievement, that, at this stage, we can experience pride and pleasure in the way we have lived and the things we have achieved; a relief and release in having passed the struggles and striving which marked younger years, and a realization of what, as a result of things learned, we are now capable of doing. Phyllis Fairley, in her late forties, expresses real exuberance: 'It is wonderful to grow older gracefully and have the growing confidence that it brings. You are more content with life as the urgency seems to grow less and you are able to relax more. You have gained more knowledge and are able to converse on many more subjects. You accept more and worry less about what others think of you; you mellow. All these are pluses.'

For Barry Jenks, now fifty, there is a relief in the place he has reached: 'I no longer feel worried that I will be shown up as unable to do certain things. I have a sense of who I am, I know my strengths and limitations. I'm nothing like as neurotic as I used to be.' But even here the measuring of gain comes with recognition that mid-life is, in Phyllis' words: 'a two-edged sword' – a time at which we recognize that the ageing process is sapping energy, closing certain doors while offering its rewards. Theoretically many of us can see that there is much good about what lies ahead if we can keep faith in ourselves and set about seeing the positive things that later life offers. In the chapter 'Looking Forward', I shall consider how the post mid-life years may indeed be an altogether more rewarding and spirited time than many of us at mid-life can imagine.

Yet the disturbing and confusing hallmark of mid-life is that, like the pattern in a kaleidoscope given a vigorous shake, the good feelings can shift suddenly and dramatically. American psychologist Mark Gerzon, based in California (the land where mid-life has been labelled 'the M-word'), was led by his own despair at his conflicting feelings to write a very personal book about the mid-life experience. He inveighs against the attitudes which he believes led to his own crisis point. 'In America we were all in love with staying young. That works until a certain point in life. But if you only love what's young, eventually you'll start to hate yourself.' So there is the perplexing situation of a sign pointing you clearly to the exit gate from youth as you reach mid-life and at the same time, for Gerzon as for a good many others, recognition that the abilities and skills gained in the first half of life and the ending of certain responsibilities around this time, open the door to new possibilities. He puts it this way: 'I had a war going on inside me between the voice that said you're finished growing, you're done and another voice that said you've only begun to explore what life is about.'

In these words Gerzon suggests the way I too have felt – still feel, indeed – as my psyche seems at sudden, unpredictable times, to play tug o' war with my composure. There is the seemingly schizoid shift between a thoroughly gratifying and enjoyable confidence which has come through survival and success in work and as a mother, as well as a greater feeling of peace with myself than I had during the restless uncertainty of my youthful days. There is a delight in friendships which have weathered and, indeed, strengthened through through the years and which I see as offering much for the future. But then these virtues of maturity are powerfully pushed aside by the shock of realizing how many experiences are passed and cannot be re-lived, that ageing means a loss of much that I have enjoyed in being young and that has felt integral to the person I believe I am. Like the playwright Hugh Whitemore, I still feel a youngster inside, but the world outside informs me that I am not viewed or valued that way. There are times when, with a kind of frenetic desperation, I believe I should radically change all the things in my life which often feel nurturing and satisfying and try to live life a new way before it is too late.

Not everybody, as I have already said, goes through this turbulence, but my interest here is in exploring mid-life as it is for the very many who do perceive it as a critical time; those who wish to understand more of why this should be so and to realize that it is not a random, individual aberrance, but that they are in considerable company.

One thing is sure, whether we like it or not mid-life is happening. A quarter of Europeans and 21 per cent of Americans are now going through the middle years. By the year 2000 people over forty will make up one in four of the EC's population, while middle-aged Americans will outnumber pre-teens by more than two to one.

As we reach this state it can be particularly unnerving to feel that we have lost our identity, that the persona which has worked thus far, no longer seems to fit. Journalist Cindy Anderson, reflecting on this in her forties, describes it vividly: 'Everyone knows what young people are like; everyone knows what old people are like. What the hell are middle-aged people supposed to be like? I don't know the script . . . I don't know the play . . . all I know is that I am not yet decrepit enough for Mantovani but too long in the tooth for Nirvana.'

The difficult realization that we are changing, that mid-life is not just a continuation of younger life, but a new life-stage and one which is going to challenge our certainties, comes to us in different ways. It may be the soft-footed demons arriving, almost without us realizing, to fiddle quietly with our equilibrium, or it may be *Sturm und Drang* so that we are caught in a maelstrom of turbulent emotions. There may be discomforting questions jabbling and jangling with tormenting insistence in our brains, or a wilful, preposterous compulsion to create havoc with our lives for the sake of excitement. All of these and other permutations have been described in the conversations I have had.

Simone de Beauvoir's dread of ageing led her to write an impressive study considering how the elderly have been treated in other cultures and eras, as well as considering current 'deeply ambivalent' attitudes towards the ageing. She saw mid-life as different from other key stages and she analysed much of the confusion around it as arising because we are not yet experiencing old age or engaging with its challenges, but we are forced to live in anticipation of it as a time which is thoroughly overshadowed by our beliefs in what it will be like. De Beauvoir took this hard, declaring: 'Old age looms ahead like a calamity,' while Turgenev, rather as pop stars have talked and sung of wanting to die before they are old, asked: 'Do you know the worst of all vices? It's being over fifty-five.' But there is little to beat the raw anguish of Dorothy Parker who apparently took her youthful gamine beauty as a licence to behave irresponsibly and at times abominably. She found ageing unbearable. It was the word 'middle' in 'middle-age' that triggered her angst, biographer Marion Meade tells us, because she saw it as branding her a frump. Parker at first saw skipping her fifties and getting to the seventies and eighties as the answer, declaring: 'People ought to be one of two things, young or old.' Then she realized that would scarcely be an improvement and amended it: 'No: what's the point of fooling? People ought to be one of two things, young or dead.'

It is very often at mid-life that people – but most often women – realize how little they have built for themselves in life because they have been so busy concentrating on the needs of others, and this usually means family. Many women will recognize themselves in Doris Lessing's definitive mid-life novel

The Summer Before the Dark, where Kate has devoted her
adult life to the needs of husband and children, keeping so
quiet about her own needs that nobody – even she in the end –
recognizes that they exist. It is at the time when her children
will soon leave home, her husband is ever more absorbed in
work, that Kate surveys her life: 'She could look forward to
nothing much but a dwindling away from full household
activity into getting old . . . What was she going to experience?
Nothing much more than, simply, she grew old: that successor
and repetition of the act of growing up.'

Laura, a Dutch mother of two and part-time worker, in her
mid-forties, is saying something quite similar when she rails
against the feeling that she has had the vibrant part of her life
and that being middle-aged has 'outlawed' her from ever being
a part of the heart and soul of what goes on. She puts it this
way: 'I see myself as in the suburbia of life.' Janet Burroway, a
contributor to a book of essays on women's feelings in the
middle years, found that her own changing state and status set
up a painful internal frustration: 'In my middle forties I went
through a period of two years in which I would wake and
rage. The fury was unpredictable in its target. There was
always something to attach it to – an imagined slight, a real
injustice, an irremediable wound from the past . . .'

One of the hardest aspects of mid-life can be the realization
that our looks are slipping away, that there is an inexorable
process of change into something we do not want to recognize.
It is eloquently expressed by M. F. K. Fisher's heroine in her
story 'Answer in the Affirmative': 'I was, in spite of myself,
thinking of my large bones, my greying hair, my occasional
deep weariness at being forty years old and harassed as most
forty-year-old women are by overwork, too many bills, outmoded clothes . . . I thought that I had gained some pounds
lately . . . I was turning slothful, I was slumping, I was neglect-
ing my fine femaleness . . . I was fat, and I was tired and old,
and when had it happened? Just those few years ago, I had
been slender, eager, untwisted by fatigue.'

For men the greatest distress is usually less about a changing perception of the physical being (although certainly plenty of men *do* feel strongly about this as will be examined later), than about realizing that the world outside is changing its perception of us. The way we look informs how we are judged as personalities.

Children's illustrator and author Maurice Sendak, in his late sixties, looks out on to the yellow gold autumn view from his Connecticut home, a place where years blend into each other in a measured routine, tranquil and purposeful, so that he is not particularly aware of time passing. He recalls how it took the arrival of a young interviewer to jolt him into uncomfortable realization: 'When I used to do a book tour or interviews I was called a hot head, a rebel, all words associated with vigorous youth. Now I am a curmudgeon and a codger, and I thought: How dare they? I mean I feel the same as ever. There was this young woman reporter who walked in and said I disappointed her because there I was, this fuming old codger – not what she expected from my books.'

It can be a solitary process, a recognition that occurs in the interior world. One man in his fifties described his feelings as: 'Looking over the precipice and seeing nothing that I could recognize or that seemed in any way what I would want. I seemed to have reached the end of time that made any sense.' Another said: 'It has happened in the past three years, I find myself tormented when somebody refers to "a bright young man" or someone who is "a high flier for his age" because I realize that no matter what I do, what talents and abilities I display, I will never be seen as a bright young man, I'll only ever be old George who hasn't done badly, has he? On those occasions I feel, quite literally, as though I'm disintegrating.'

Such feelings do not make mid-life feel like an important life-stage, a time when we are limbering up to do some significant psychological growing, and when the most painful feelings may in fact be a kind of growing pain, yet the writings of many of the pre-eminent theorists and analysts in human behaviour believe this is precisely what it is. They argue, as we shall see, that the critical times we experience frequently act as a developmental kick up the backside. Mid-life can be seen as the bridge which links the place where we belonged to the young and the new terrain of the elders, and our task is to negotiate this bridge in order to arrive feeling in harmony with oneself at the other side. If we can do this, if we can use the mid-life period to make a constructive transition, then we may well experience older age as a positive time.

If we fail to do so and strive to be indistinguishable from our juniors, our knuckles white with the effort of clutching the rail at the beginning of the bridge, in the hope that we may not have to cross it and can deny what is happening, then the experience of ageing and being old may be a struggle.

The phenomenon of mid-life as just that, a mid-way point in life is a modern one. Five hundred years ago average life expectancy was the twenties and at the turn of the century the fifties, but for today's mid-lifers the average has gone well over seventy, and increasingly people are living to eighty, ninety and one hundred. So for us, the bulge-and-boom generations, mid-life has a very different meaning from that which it had for earlier generations who effectively moved from the years of adulthood in which they grew up, worked, married, had children and watched them become independent and leave the family confines, into what was seen as old age, the time leading to death.

Do we celebrate the fact that when we reach mid-life we may well have at least as much life left to live again? Do we see possibilities, opportunities for new experiences, learning new skills, developing new facets of ourselves in ways which would not have been possible earlier? Or do we see it more as a life-sentence, a lot of years rendered null and void in a society where ageism and discrimination have led to a bleak array of attitudes and feelings around getting older, reflected in the line of writer Anthony Powell: 'Growing old is like being increasingly penalized for a crime you haven't committed.'

But why should it be this way? As already touched upon, the young were interesting economically after teenagers were invented in the 1950s; equally and quite understandably they appeared, after the darkness of the war years, to offer the possibility for transformation and change. They were the new generation who would somehow make the world seem a brave new place. In this enthusiastic climate they became leaders of the pack: their clothes, their music, their tastes, their ideas on life became the thing to follow. Youth became the gold standard and whereas cultural fashions usually live out a limited span and change, the cult of youth hung on and on. Ever since Twiggy set a fashion for models who looked scarcely out of Babygros, we've had virtually pre-pubescent kids being deified on the catwalk; a few old musicians have shown their faces and swung their hips, and continue to do so, but the favourite flavour remains close to the nursery. In the workplace the young are seen to have freshness, a cutting edge, ideas that nobody who has been around, learning the ropes, notching up expertise and a knowledge of what is going on, can apparently match. And when it comes to sex ... well, nubile young curves, or boyish biceps remain the definition of desirable.

A major player in all this is, of course, advertising which has left us in no doubt about young being the best seller, and over and over my interview subjects spoke out about how angry it makes them to be either blanked out from depictions of the world they live in in advertisements, or portrayed almost exclusively in ads for laxatives and sheepskin slippers.

While television critic Allison Pearson relates how, even for documentaries about real life, she has heard producers deciding not to use someone because she explains: 'They look a bit old or are a bit stumbling and not "good telly". So although they represent reality, they are barred from making a contribution unless it's a programme about granny battering or Britain's poor old folk, then the more decrepit they look the more they are welcomed.' When they do appear centre stage it is in a range of stereotypes: quaint old dears, spirited golden oldies and joyless curmudgeons – Victor Meldrew has a lot to answer for in perpetuating our collective fear of ending up as a version of him. The press is scarcely better, using euphemisms like: 'wonderful for her age'; 'still got all his marbles'; and 'wonderfully well preserved'.

To recognize how thoroughly the youth factor has penetrated our way of seeing risks sounding like sour grapes when it comes from one who is, so to speak, the wrong side of the tracks. But it is not intended this way. Indeed my generation has benefited from obsessive youth culture and we have to acknowledge our own complicity in it. Nor is looking at how powerfully the idea that young is almost always the best flavour intended as an attack on the young. The present young have not created this value system, nor is life all that easy for them – interestingly while mid-lifers may envy certain aspects of youth, and wish they were available to them in their present life-stage, few say they would actually want to BE young living a youngster's life today.

The point is that valuing youth should not mean negating age. Yet that is precisely what it has progressively meant in the post-war years. We rarely see older or even middle-aged people represented as equalling the young for interest value or living a vibrant lifestyle.

Indeed the image of ageing is sufficiently bad that a British survey reported in the early 1990s that a substantial number of people as young as thirty-five dreaded getting old, while Age Concern in their survey of one thousand people from eleven-year-olds to those over sixty-five, found largely negative expectations of old age. Similar findings come from America. Nearly one in three of those interviewed for Age Concern expect older people to be grumpy and mean. Sixteen per cent expected to be sad and lonely in old age and a further 15 per cent believed society sees older people as slow and doddery. In societies that have become increasingly inhuman in their pursuit of product, efficiency and independence from state help, the elderly have seen their standing diminish. Author Jeanette Kupferman regards the way the elderly are now treated as a reflection of a disposable society where, she suggests, the machine paradigm of the body has bred the idea that: 'The old and less efficient apparatus must be scrapped and replaced with a new and more efficient model.' No wonder the elderly have come to feel horribly close to American writer Art Linkletter's observation of man's four stages as: 'Infancy, childhood, adolescence and obsolescence.'

It is a terrible indictment of a society that it makes us feel this way, and how different growing old might be if there were role and ritual to reward us, to demonstrate society's veneration as we notch up the years of experience, and if in return we were given the opportunity to offer services which were valued as the product of our years lived. Imagine if we lived in one of those societies both past and present where Donald Cowgill, examining ageing in different societies, describes 'an individual's life as a continuous progression', and explains how each transition represents a movement towards greater responsibility and higher status. In such cultures, he says, old age is the pinnacle of life, the ultimate achievement. In Mozambique the eldest male in a lineage is chosen as 'father of the people' to speak to the ancestral spirits in times of famine. Among the Sidamo of Ethiopia, an elder, when she becomes a grandmother, may demand that a grandchild be given to her to be raised as a personal servant, and as she becomes the eldest in the village she will be put in charge of organizing housewarmings and harvest rituals. Older women in some pre-industrial tribes are in charge of the practice of tattooing while older men may be chosen to do scarifying and nose perforation for the initiation ceremonies of the young. Women, too, often assume the valued task of midwife as they age – their life's experience is seen to qualify them.

If mid-life were in effect the time of preparation for the tasks and responsibilities conferred on us by age, it would surely feel very different. Perhaps there would be less of the distress voiced by writer Martin Amis: 'Nothing had prepared me for the unqualified nightmare of early middle-age.' He went on to leave a wife and two children for a younger woman.

But in our society we have no recognition of accrued responsibility to give mid-life a meaning we can value. Far from being presented to us as a stage of significance, mid-life is treated as limboland. To be middle-aged is, apparently, to be nowhere in particular with no real purpose. It is a time reduced *en passant* to jokey regret at the spreading waistline and the disappearing hair, the subject of Brighton beach postcards where leery old men conspicuously past their prime make crude remarks about blonde hourglass bimbos.

There is something absurd about mid-life – the time when we have gained the knowledge and confidence from decades spent living, and when most people are still physically active and mentally involved in the world they live in – having no meaning, nor indeed having even commanded the interest and analysis which other stages in our development have. Gail Sheehy in her study of life's stages talks of mid-life as the least researched, least thought-out aspect of our existence: 'The apostrophe in time between the end of growing up and beginning of growing old,' while Gerzon, recalling his sense of futility and hollowness when mid-life hit and he had no idea how to make sense of his existence, talks angrily of: 'the black hole of the human life cycle'.

The problem is that we have no preparation for mid-life. There is no decent map to suggest a good route, or warn us against the worst swamps and savagery. Instead we embark on this new terrain, stumbling and thrashing, trying to carve a path. The first half of life has a well defined map with a clear-cut set of goals, aspirations and tasks laid out for us as we become adults, so that even if we do not succeed in achieving them they at least provide us with a framework for a way of living, or conventions and expectations to rebel against.

The years when we grow from childhood to young adult-hood, are signposted with a great deal of information and guidance along the way. We are given the tools we need to cope, the knowledge that will help us, warned about the pitfalls we may encounter. But then the clear markings on our life-map seem to fade out, diminishing to a few higgledy-piggledy minor roads. We find we are on our own.

Laurence Hughes is in his mid-forties and has four children to support from a small picture-framing business he runs. There was little time during the earlier years to stop and contemplate what he was doing with life or whether it matched up to his expectations. He clutches a large china mug between his hands, his face a study of uncertainty: 'Everything had seemed clear cut, there were things to be done and ways to do them – more or less – throughout my thirties but when I hit my forties nothing looked straightforward any more. I could see that the tools I had been using to deal with life were not the right tools for the next part. But I didn't know what tools I needed and I felt so scared, so bereft of the person I had been who seemed to know what to do with his life.'

Magda Breen, a literary agent in her late forties, has seen herself as an explorer standing at the edge of an open space and she says: 'I realize I have to work out a way for myself, that I must find my own way to get around the boulders, across the hidden clumps of grass which might trip me, through the sudden patches of dark growth which will not part and let me see the way through. It is a daunting prospect but I can also see that it might be exciting. I am growing daily more used to the idea that I am not a young woman any more and I shan't be again and I don't feel I have any idea what that means.'

It is the sense of being alone, that perhaps there is something amiss about our lack of sure-footedness at this stage; our questioning. the feeling that we need to change things but quite possibly don't know what needs changing or how to do it, which is daunting. Are we alone in this state? Should we do all within our power to ignore it and go on as ever? Or should we follow what may seem a wayward inclination? They are puzzling and disturbing questions, as many people talking with me have acknowledged. But so many people who feel this way tend not to say it because they do not easily admit to anything which may represent weakness or lack of adequacy. How much easier it might be if there were some sort of preparation, planning even, for mid-life.

M. F. K. Fisher voiced this view: 'Parts of the ageing process are scary of course, but the more we know about them, the less they need be. That is why I wish we were more deliberately taught, in early years, to prepare for this condition.'

Carl Jung, who was intensely interested in the ways we may make positive transitions in later life, understood the dilemma well: 'Wholly unprepared we embark upon the second half of life ... thoroughly unprepared we take the step into the afternoon of life, worse still, we take this step with the false assumption that our truths and ideas will serve as hitherto. But we cannot live the afternoon of life according to the pro-gramme of life's morning.' This is, of course, the point. We have to understand and accept that we need to devise a schema which is appropriate to the physical and mental changes which must take place, that we must find a way of valuing what our years passed mean rather than regretting what is lost. For if we attempt to live a later life that is an increasingly thin and desperate shadow of younger life, we will certainly live by the law of diminishing returns.

Jung has written at length about this as something which we must do by learning to see that letting go of youth and living as an elder is, in fact, progress and can lead to a rewarding later life. But he explained, it means doing something which I, among many, have found to be an ongoing challenge – finding a way to see that the competitive, constantly active, demanding way of life so many of us develop during our first half of life, does not make for good living in the second half. The most likely scenario if we do this is that we will become increasingly dejected and exhausted. This is not to say that we have to give up on all the things we have enjoyed doing, but rather that we need to try to pull away from the quest for external approval, a place in the limelight, the striving for opportunities which are given to the young, and learn to cultivate satisfaction and pleasure in a more quietly creative way, and one that allows us to be comfortable with ourselves and to leave space for spiritual growth.

The Hindus see it as self-evident that we need some kind of defining experience to prepare us for older age, and that spiritual growth is a *sine qua non* of this. They believe that as the script appears to end at forty it is only sensible to have a crisis and discover what the purpose is for the rest of your life. But whereas in Western cultures we strive to blot out mental and physical pain as best we can, so that there is little place for spiritual development, in many Eastern cultures they see life as a process of learning, acceptance, stoicism and tranquillity.

Therapist Kenne Zugman who works with male executives from Silicone Valley in California – men who tend to want clear-cut problem-solving programmes – has drawn inspiration from Eastern philosophies. So when these captains of industry reach his consulting room because, Zugman explains, 'the centre does not seem to be holding', they are usually looking for a practical answer to what is wrong. He says: 'I have to explain to them that there is no twelve-point plan which will sort out the fact they feel empty, that nothing makes sense, their marriages seem to have lost meaning. I suggest that they need to find a way to stop and take stock of their lives and perhaps re-cast the way they are living so that the future seems to offer a vision they can bear or even anticipate with pleasure.'

He goes on to explain that: 'If mid-life is proving difficult then I regard that as a clear signal that we should be examining our lives and our attitudes to getting older. It *IS* frightening. I feel frightened, I believe everyone does at some level because what we are talking about is finite time. But the great advantage to being a grown up is that we have probably learned a few skills and if we put our mind to it, we can use these to guide us.'

Accepting that youth has passed may require a ritual. Sue Landesworth, a seamstress in her early fifties, has had a succession of dreams in which she wore a red dress that was to be taken away. She sees this as symbolic of going through the menopause, the aspect of mid-life which she found most thoroughly forced her to face the loss of youth. She says: 'I knew that if I didn't stop wanting to be young so that time was passing in a state of dissatisfaction, sadness and anger at knowing I was asking the impossible, I would go on suffering and being destructive. So I forced myself to mourn my youth, to see myself as someone who had achieved something in moving on from it. I forced myself to think about my daughter and her youth and I thought a lot about how my life had been at that age, how I had enjoyed my youth and in an almost ceremonial way I told myself it was dead and to be buried.

'Of course nothing is quite so simple but I did feel I'd made a psychological breakthrough in being clear I was ready to move on from my fixation with being young.'

The way George chose to make mid-life what he regards as a thoroughly constructive time, was by taking 'my somewhat dishevelled body in hand and exercising until I thought I'd explode then feeling terrific afterwards. It gave me a great sense of powerfulness and I went on to run a demanding race in my late fifties. I went on a Saga holiday which was enormous fun and I was one of the youngest – the kid! Then I joined a tennis club and a singles set-up so that suddenly my middle years were busy and rewarding, and the fact that I'd been usurped by a younger man at work – very much the cause of a nosedive I took in my late forties – seemed to matter a great deal less. In fact I was glad not to be having to work all the hours God gave me and always taking a briefcase home.'

My aim in exploring how we may find ourselves puzzled, questioning and uncertain at mid-life has been to suggest that this transitional time should not be seen just as a meaningless staging post in our existence. But the thing we need to grasp and remember while stepping off on our journey into the next part of life is that it is an individual and often quite solitary one. We might wish for a clearly defined route, a set format for dealing with whatever issues we face, but the point is that we have to work things through and learn how to grow in a way that suits each of us according to who we are. Author Wayne Booth put it well, saying: 'We can't reach old age by another man's road. My habits protect my life but they would assassinate you.'

Old, Moi?

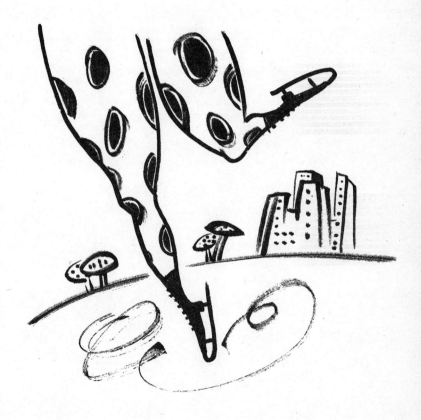

Like a white candle
In a holy place,
So is the beauty
Of an aged face . . .
JOSEPH CAMPBELL, '*The Old Woman*'

IT IS IN THE MIRROR that we are brought face to face with mid-life; the uncompromising reflection offering a steady progress report as we pass through the time zones. In this intimate encounter we see how irrevocably the ageing process is making itself known. We see the crinkles and crumples, the lines and bags under the eyes. We may find as Gipsy Rose Lee did that: 'I have everything now I had twenty years ago – except it's all lower.' No matter how well we look after ourselves, how kind nature may be, as we reach the middle years we will be aware that changes have occurred that, like pictures manipulated on a computer screen, can prefigure how we may appear in older age.

Yet what we see is not just the process of entropy, but the marks of our history, the events we have lived through. Our faces are a measure of the lives we have lived: there may be laughter lines and the deeper furrows caused by stress or sadness; there may be bags under the eyes from the rigours of bringing up children, of working hard, of living energetically. Shouldn't we then celebrate the fact that we have done so much, that we have played our part in the world? Lynne Kirkham, just turning forty thinks so, and her feisty, combative attitude is cheering: 'Most people even in old age can be attractive, interesting and fun to be with. An older confident person who obviously enjoys life often radiates a more subtle but deeper beauty. But sexual beauty seems to be an obsession at the moment.'

It would be nice if we could all say as actress Sheila Hancock did with wonderful brio: 'I've earned every one of these wrinkles and I'm proud of them,' but in truth most of us are far more inclined to be as harsh and hard on ourselves as Wicksteed in Alan Bennett's play *Habeas Corpus* who, albeit humorously, describes himself as a 'worn defeated fool'. And to echo the sentiments of the 17th-century French beauty and courtesan Ninon de Lenclos: 'If God had to give a woman wrinkles He might at least have put them on the soles of her feet.' In other words we may feel pride in what we have done, the personalities we have become through the years, but we do not care for the signs of it writ large.

I experience this ambiguity myself. I take pride in the fact that I have brought up two sons who seem to me people worth sending out into the world, that I have put effort into work I consider worthwhile, that I have struggled to build and maintain relationships and friendships. And yet the visible legacy of the years spent doing this does not give me pleasure. I resent the loss of a clear, taut young skin, the sight of some grey hairs, the mosaic of crinkles on the back of my hands, and I hear a great many of my contemporaries, men and women, expressing similar sentiments.

One reason, surely, is that we feel we are failing when we age, that somehow we have not been smart enough to avoid letting it happen, and that is the legacy of living in what writer Germaine Greer has called a 'youthist culture', which tells us very clearly that our value shrinks with every visible year. The point is neatly made on a contemporary birthday card depicting an oldish woman saying: 'They tell me getting older means I have wisdom and character . . . but I'd rather have a cute ass!'

There are people whose lives are sufficiently contented or successful that they claim not to be worried by mid-life or the prospect of becoming old, but my research suggests that far more people are without this sense of certainty. Almost every argument I have heard making a positive or even sanguine case for the loss of youthful looks sounds at best *faute de mieux* and more often like the hollow howl of defiant rationalization.

So it is that as we reach the middle years the mirror assumes a symbolic meaning. We are constantly aware of its existence, knowing that it is the medium with the message we are loath to receive. Ava Gardner, an actress who, in my view, matured with beauty and sensuality, could not bear what she saw when she looked for reassurance in the looking glass and suggested: 'All beautiful women should smash their mirrors early.'

But she missed the point, as did Emily Carr, even though she neatly pinned the dilemma when she wrote: 'It is the ugliness of old age I hate. Being old is not bad if you keep away from mirrors.' Even if we resolutely turn our eyes from any reflected image of ourselves, we know we are ageing, we know how ageing is regarded in society, we know that whether we see what is happening or not, the world around us sees the truth and reflects it back in the way we are looked at, spoken to and treated.

Journalist Brenda Polan's experience is echoed by both men and women: 'The mornings I wake having had a few glasses of wine the night before and stayed up late, I look at all this drooping flesh in the mirror and think I hate it, that's not fair, that's not me, that's not what I want to be. It's all happening too quickly and I never bargained for it to happen so soon.'

Alistair Mead, a financial adviser in his early fifties, expresses the shock of learning what passing time has meant: 'I came across a photo of myself, in my thirties, the other day and realized just how much I have changed and aged. I'm not a great one for too much close encountering with my face in the mirror except when I'm shaving, and then all I see is the soap and the stubble. But after seeing the photo I went and had a good hard look in the mirror and I realized that no matter what I did I would never look as I had in my early thirties, again. It depressed me, if I'm honest.'

The reflection in the mirror taunts Phyllis Fairley with a physical self that seems at odds with what she feels she has achieved as a person: 'It seems unjust to have the confidence of maturity with a sagging body.'

And why should it be otherwise? If, from earliest years we learn that beauty or handsomeness equals youth, is it surprising that we find it hard to believe there can be value in the look of later years?

All the more so for those whose identities that have been built around youthful looks, because they are most prone to a sense of disintegration and uselessness. Lauren Hutton, whose successful career as a model was built on a clear-faced wholesome beauty, nosedived most painfully at the age of forty-five. She conceptualized the rejection by her profession in the form of harshly judgmental mirrors: 'I felt I was bottoming out. I had stopped looking at *Vogue*. It was painful to always see very young girls because you compare yourself to them. The world of modelling is like being surrounded by mirrors and they are the outside world judging you.'

Yet Lauren's tale is ultimately a redemptive one, for it was after this crisis time, just as she was reaching fifty, that Steven Meisel, described as the young photographer of the moment, asked Hutton if she would do an advertising campaign for an American department store. He spelled out the particular appeal Hutton, as an older woman, had for him: 'I was fascinated by her modernness and style. And she was extremely sexy – especially at that age. There's more to photograph with a woman than with a little girl.' The advertising campaign not only resuscitated Hutton's career but turned her into a heroine so that women would come up to her on the street and thank her for rescuing them from invisibility.

Actor Harvey Keitel is a different but as cheering an example of a public face which has come into its own with ageing. The erstwhile chubby, bad-boy-on-the-block look so familiar in the early Martin Scorsese films has matured, and as his looks have become more craggy and lined they have also become more interesting, sensitive, and sensual. Many women lusted over him in his role as the middle-aged *enfant sauvage* in Jane Campion's film *The Piano*, even though his exposed body was a far cry from the lissom, limber frames of the more junior objects of desire.

So our assumptions may not always be correct. There is a shift in attitude towards ageing and the look of maturity which is, perhaps, not surprising when you consider that most of the young blades of the 1960s who set standards in taste and style are now mid-lifers, and they are influential in the image-making industries. It is not surprising that they are using their corporate skills to spread the idea that middle-age is a good place to be. It has become almost commonplace for newspapers and magazines to run articles pinpointing some film star, actor or business personality as a shining example of matured beauty, handsomeness or style. Model agencies have sprung to life specifically to handle women nearer the menopause than puberty, and older men too are being used in advertisements as chic sex symbols driving chic cars, for example, rather than as quaint caricatures.

An extraordinarily successful example of popular culture putting across the idea that mid-lifers are not just good enough, but better than that, is Robert James Waller's novel *The Bridges of Madison County* which became a bestseller first in America then across the world. It is the tale of two middle-aged characters who are presented in a way which suggests they are desirable, attractive, sensual:

The first serious lines were just beginning to show on her face . . . Still, she was pleased with what she saw. Her hair was black, and her body was full and warm, filling out the jeans just about right . . . He was thin and hard . . . his grey hair was long and dishevelled . . . He wasn't handsome, not in any conventional sense. But there was something about him. Something very old, something slightly battered by the years.

The important point about this is that the characters Francesca Johnson in her mid-forties and Robert Kincaid in his fifties are drawn to each other *because* of, not in spite of, the fact that the way they look reflects maturity. Waller has made the point that in Francesca's filled out body, the serious lines, and Robert's battered look, they recognize a width of experience, a depth of emotion which would be missing without the years lived. Age does not detract from physical beauty and sensuality here but gives it a different dimension.

But however cheering these signs of change may be, they are of the moment, while the things today's mid-life generations are grappling with are attitudes and feelings moulded by the times we have grown up in and which form the basis of our beliefs and psychological conditioning. Although we have the benefits of much knowledge and some products which can help us prevent ourselves ageing as fast as other generations have, both in appearance and health, I do not believe that we will come to terms with the look of ageing and move forward to play our part in creating a new older aesthetic, until we understand how powerfully our strings are pulled by underlying forces.

So it is that when my teenage son, who has not seen my partner and me for several months, remarks one evening that he can see how his father and I have aged, I feel demolished. Why do we – for I know my partner also takes it hard – find it so painful to hear this judgment, and why does it make us feel diminished, so much less than it did when he used to tell us how young his friends thought we looked?

The answer is that we have been part of those generations growing up with ageism spreading and seeping into many aspects of life, so that, even though we may see examples of mid-lifers and older-looking people who are attractive and well cared for in a way we admire, it does not register as having value in the way youth does. Our identities are intimately tied up with how we look which means that if we have lived in a culture which rewards and applauds us for our youthful looks, but then ceases to be interested, effectively rendering us invisible as we age, then it is as though our whole identity is being negated.

Pamela Maclaren, in her fifties, has had a hard life bringing up four children on a low income and seeing her husband through several affairs before leaving him, and she feels a certain bitterness at having coped with that and being rewarded at the end of doing what she regards as a valuable job with the loss of 'my selling power'. She says: 'I used to be a cute little thing – that's what I was told – and like it or not, it was my looks that opened doors, got me opportunities, made people listen to the garbage I spoke a lot of the time.

'What I've got inside now is much richer, much better than that. I know the world, I have real wisdom about human behaviour. I know about how kids tick, I know how to survive. But who cares? I don't represent the best sweeties in the bag so I'm not worth anything. That's how I feel.'

Will Bullen, a homeopathist in his late forties, says: 'When I was young I got a lot of interest and attention from women and men. It seemed that my looks drew people to me and made them interested in me. My hair has thinned in the past few years and because I've worked in hot climates a good deal I'm pretty weathered – well wrinkled – and I probably look older than I am. I have done a lot and I am told I am an interesting companion, but I am very well aware that I don't get the attention I used to.'

A way of seeing that denies maturity and makes a fetish of youth turns the ageing physique into something which can all too easily be despised by its owner. That comes through poignantly in the words of fifty-seven-year-old Anne Vanderschoot: 'I miss so very much the beauty of youth and quite honestly I don't think I will ever come to terms with it. I hate what ageing is doing to my skin. I have always been proud of my looks and worked hard to keep my skin and hair in good condition; my weight stays steady because of careful eating. I still wear make up and wear smart and stylish clothes and yet it is a losing battle because nature catches up and all the hard work seems in vain. Will I always look with envy at my daughter's beautiful skin? I hope not but at the moment I do.'

The sense that the look of age makes us invisible comes up so often. The anguish and fury of Catherine Howard at the way she believes the look of an aged face and body alters everything, is palpable: 'Middle-aged women get used to being called "an old bag". Street canvassers ignore us, the theory being that we now have neither brains, money nor opinions worth canvassing. Young mothers with pushchairs are the most aggressive in the hate campaign against the grey-haired agilely-disadvantaged female.

'My local off-licence has a wine-tasting session every Saturday. If I stood there with a basketful of fivers and my tongue hanging out until closing time, I would not be offered a glass. I am one of the great invisibles.'

It was a shock for Shirley Anne Field, an actress in her late forties, whose loveliness is often remarked upon and who is used to being highly visible, to learn how instantly the look of ageing eclipses that prominence. When filming *Lady Chatterley's Lover*, in which she played the ageing housekeeper, she became sharply aware of the eyes passing over her when she finished filming but remained in the plain dress and with an unmade-up face – the appearance she needed for her part. She talked poignantly of how it made her feel she did not exist.

Men may frame the feelings they have differently, and there are reasons, as will be discussed later, why the issue has different meaning for men and women, but it can nevertheless affect them deeply too.

Californian Huey Goldschmidt, a store salesman in his mid-fifties, talks of his experience: 'There is this increasing awareness that people's eyes go over you and do not want to see you as you age, and it is a direct correlation with the number of lines appearing on the face, the hair greying, skin sagging. When I was in my twenties and I walked into a bookstore or coffee bar I was aware of being looked at, of being highly visible. As I get older, people look past me to the young, hard bodies and I am forced against all my wishes to see that I don't exist in the same way. I see the twenty-year-old, but the twenty-year-old doesn't see me. It's very painful because I feel there's nothing I can do or be to make myself visible again.'

There is, of course, nothing new in the deification of youth and its equation with beauty, or in the abhorrence of the signs of ageing. Writers, poets, philosophers, artists through the ages have expressed this perspective. Wayne Booth (*The Art of Growing Older*) has gathered together a few of the adjectives used by the Romans to describe those deemed past their prime: 'pot-bellied; of damnable shape; flabby, loose-lipped; worn-out'.

Over and over Shakespeare expressed what was, presumably, a reflection of prevailing values when he bewailed the loss of beauty in the ageing. Take the sonnet in which he wistfully refers to 'thy beauty's field' then anticipates it will be reduced to 'a tattered weed of small worth', once forty winters have done their work. Poet Matthew Arnold talked of growing old as the loss of 'the glory of the form, the lustre of the eye', while Robert Graves saw 'Grey haunted eyes . . . cheeks, furrowed . . . teeth, few'.

And although men, because of their greater power both historically and in contemporary times, have had the opportunity to select younger women and discard those seen as past their prime, they too have at times been made to realize that age makes them less desirable. John Crowe Ransom in his poem 'Piazza Piece' tells poignantly of the older man attempting to court a young woman who shoos him away declaring: 'I am a lady young in beauty waiting.'

One timeless reason for this loathing is that it spells out the inevitability of old age and mortality. When we see an ageing face, when we see the skull beneath the skin, we are forced to recognize that we too will come to this. And if fears of mortality were bad enough in ages past, the taboo on death has reached hysterical proportions in the West this past half-century – so much so that in America a group called the Immortalists have convinced themselves that, with sufficient will-power, they can defy death. The effect on us as we age and feel the antipathy towards what we have become, is not just that we are no longer seen as youngsters, but that we may no longer be lovable.

The American poet Nilene O.A. Foxworth has expressed these fears in a way that could, equally, be said on behalf of a man:

> 'Will you love me when I'm old
> When my eyelids sink behind my skull
> When my gawky gums send a trembling voice . . .
> When I am arid as the desert
> And my firm breast sags
> Like an old laundry bag.

But today's mid-lifers have more to battle against than centuries before have had if they are to combat ageism and make acceptable the look of age. Communities have fragmented and changed their basic structure, so that whereas in the past it was likely that extended families lived close, that elderly people were part of a neighbourhood where generations had grown up and they had a valued role in caring for and sharing their families' young, that role is less likely to exist today.

Furthermore, the West has built youth and beauty up to have mythical significance in the post-war years, and the belief that how we look will dictate our value in life begins almost at birth with beautiful baby contests, little Miss Pears competitions, events which pitch pubescent girls against each other, teaching that she with the loveliest curves, the best head of hair, is a winner. And increasingly young men are being taught to worship the body beautiful, rolling up for events where they flex over-developed muscles hoping to be voted Mr-something-marvellous. But all this stops abruptly by the time we approach mid-life.

A clear line has been drawn between the young presented for our consumption in styles and poses which emphasize how youthful or childlike they are, or described in print with salivating adjectives and a kind of breathless wonder, a glorying in what American psychologist Rita Freedman, in her analysis of the beauty industry describes as their neotenic traits: 'neo meaning new, tein meaning to stretch – literally the look of a newborn is stretched into adulthood', and the ageing who come in for a different kind of imagery. Robert Waller's Francesca Johnson and Robert Kincaid are rare compared with how the middle-aged are so often portrayed as apologetically faded into subdued discretion like the forty-seven-year-old widow Julia Ferndale in William Trevor's *Other People's Lives*, who dares not risk a bouffant hairdo or colour rinse for fear of being labelled as mutton dressed as lamb. Or they are presented as downright unappetizing as in the style of the overweight, florid, peanut-biscuit-nibbling fifty-five-year-old Harry Angstrom in John Updike's Rabbit novel (*Rabbit at Rest*), whose dislike of his own ageing is projected into a view of Janice his wife:

He touches Janice at his side, the sweated white cotton of her tennis dress at the waist, to relieve his sudden sense of doom.

Her waist is thicker, has less of a dip, as she grows into that barrel body of women in late middle age, their legs getting skinny, their arms getting loose like cooked chicken coming off the bone.

Behind all this lies a powerful commercial imperative designed to feed off the anxiety in our collective unconscious. If we can be made to feel inadequate enough about ourselves, then we can be manipulated into buying expensive potions and lotions, techniques and methods which we hope will offset the look of age. The way it is done is by using models considerably younger, as a rule, than the ageing customer being targeted, so that our own faces, supposedly to be equated with those in the advertisements, do not match up. We buy the dream of looking the way the model does, and the dream will be blown, of course, if advertisers use someone who actually looks middle-aged. We saw, for example, how within a few short months, two mid-life women whose faces are generally agreed to be beautiful but of a certain age – Isabella Rossellini who modelled cosmetics for Lancôme and Joanna Lumley, who was used to advertise the German Müller yogurts – lost their contracts because, apparently, they were too old.

Purveyed images define and dictate our way of seeing, living proof of the view expressed by Scottish philosopher David Hume, more than two hundred years ago, that there are no universally acceptable standards. Beautiful faces are simply those which satisfy taste.

Present mid-life generations have grown up in the post-war years during which the development of technology and electronic imagery has manipulated and distorted what we see and how we see it, and has created its own selective normality. The fast-moving, scarcely glimpsed image, the perspective suggested by an elliptical picture, the advertisement that suggests in just a glimpse the rewards its product brings, are almost without exception posited on the use of very young models and performers. Television's entertainment and game shows rarely feature an older person and if they do, the supporting 'players', the fun and glamour content, will be young. Many soaps are weighted towards the exploits of the young and, one Boston psychologist observed: 'When you have a soap about a family it's often the kids as main players criticizing the older generations.'

While the young are dressed in zappy clothes and given physically and sometimes mentally taxing tasks to perform in shows like *Gladiators*, bringing admiration from many viewers, by contrast the TV game devised for 'grannies' made them into figures of fun where they were swung around in cages from which they had to be rescued.

It is known that the visual media have enormous impact on the way opinions are formed, so it is easy to see how the 'youth picture' creates an image of normality which, by omission, excludes elders. As the authors of *Ageing in Society*, a study of what it means to age in different societies, explain: 'The mass media reproduces stereotypes and circulates images at a faster pace and to a wider audience than ever before. It is now possible to close your eyes and ears to images with which you do not identify, but it is not possible to ignore the pervasive presence of images as such.'

If, then, we do not see older people as part of everyday life, as part of popular entertainment, as participating in the many ways they do in real life, along with the young, as part of the visual information which is incessantly moulding our view of the world, then they do not fit the picture of normal life. When the older face is excluded from depictions of life, because it is not considered attractive enough to draw viewers and sell products, it becomes abnormal, something which does not fit properly. For example, Joan Goodman, journalist and Hollywood commentator, points out: 'Every major part, even for people considerably older, is shown first to Michelle Pfeiffer, Tom Cruise, Brad Pitt, Sharon Stone – the film companies see them as the faces which will draw audiences.'

The significance of the young winning the bulk of the active, interesting roles where they portray important, influential characters and speak the most meaningful lines is that they have come to be seen not just as defining the best in good looks but as the most dynamic, inventive, empathetic and energetic, those who say things worth hearing. We do not have to look far to see how this has been replicated in real life in the post-war years. Job descriptions began, conspicuously, to have upper age limits and to stress the wish for youth and dynamism. Top jobs in the city went to youngsters while mature executives were moved out of the way. And something similar took root in business, in the media; bratpack writers are considered more 'sexy' than their matured counterparts; as a thirty-something film-maker said: 'These days a twenty-five-year-old artist is supposed to have done something definitive in his genre or he's seen as almost past it.' A far cry from the days when the forty-one-year-old Henry Moore was talked of as a promising young artist.

A steady shift took place from the times when experience, wisdom, and knowledge of life – the qualities we have, we hope, acquired in the first half of life during which we will presumably have tackled some major life events – were traditionally balanced against the inexperience of those whose looks came to be seen as embodying something more full of promise and possibility.

It is a situation which enrages those who declare over and over that they feel little different from the way they did twenty years ago, and are considerably more in substance than they were then. Fashion designer Katharine Hamnett expresses a widely held anger and frustration: 'I am so much more than I was as a young woman. I know how to run a successful business, I have the confidence to express views and argue the toss which must make me more entertaining company than in earlier years. I know I have learnt to be a better lover than I used to be.

'All that shows in my looks – it shows in the fact that I don't look young and unformed any longer. But that's not what counts. In our culture, broadly speaking, mind and flesh are the same thing: if the flesh doesn't look right then forget the mind.'

She contrasts this with what she has seen while journeying in the Far East: 'I am always struck by how the older people I see are in so much better shape, psychologically, than their counterparts at home. If you go to Thailand you see older people there of sixty or seventy who are so powerful because of the place they hold in their communities and that means they feel proud of who they are. It shows in their faces, that feeling creates its own beauty and dignity. They take pride in their bodies, they dress beautifully rather than hiding themselves away. Whereas in the West I see – I experience it myself – denial of what is happening and such fear of what it means to look older.'

Martin Beresford, a marketing manager in his mid-forties, feels disadvantaged in the company of younger men and says: 'I go to a seminar, a group event, a dinner party and if I see younger men I feel immediately that they will be the main players, the people who are of interest. I feel their youthful appearance draws eyes and makes people want to listen to them. I might be able to talk with far more authority than them, have had experiences they haven't, I might be a far more well-rounded personality. But I feel disadvantaged by the fact that I don't look the way the youngsters do, that somehow what I have to offer is seen as dull, pedestrian, because that's what age means.'

The way we feel as we watch the ageing process played out physically on our bodies will be exacerbated or mitigated by many things: the way we have been helped or hindered in valuing ourselves from childhood, the approval and affection we have won through our personality and actions are significant in affecting how much self-esteem we have when we reach mid-life.

The person who feels good about the way he or she has used their years, who feels valued for what they are rather than how they look, will almost certainly be better able to adjust to and accept the look of ageing better than the person who has never been able to cut free from the feeling that being young, having a youthful appearance, is integral to being liked, loved, admired, employed or any of the other things which represent practical and psychic survival. The kind of community we live in, whether we are among long-standing friends or family, how highly our skills are valued and remain so, will all have a bearing on this.

We often hear it argued that we should be able to rise above worrying over the way we look, and never more so than as we age. We are expected to have grown beyond frivolous concerns. Yet this is nonsense. There is nothing frivolous about concern with our appearance. It is endlessly hammered into us as the most serious of matters. We learn young what it means not to fit an acceptable standard. The child who does not conform to what is defined as absolute normality will know and probably suffer for it; the person with a handicap or facial deformation will never be free of society's discomforting appraisal of them. The overweight person knows well that they cannot expect to be valued as highly as somebody who fits the ideal.

In communities where there are strong prevailing standards of 'good' and 'bad', feelings of being an outsider can be particularly difficult as psychologists Ray Bull and Nichola Ramsey have found: 'Most of us have a desire to conform to the standards that we believe are the norm for our society. A failure to do so sets us aside both in our own estimation and in the estimation of others.'

The ageing face and body are not viewed as the norm, but rather as something gone wrong. Older looks do not on the whole equate with cultural ideals of beauty in the West, nor, indeed, in plenty of developing countries, but in the Third World, the elderly may be offered the compensation of additional status. Of course there are aged film stars, actors, dancers, society folk – people whose good looks have been legendary – held up from time to time with breathless delight by a newspaper or magazine as proof that you can still look terrific in spite of the passing years, but it almost always comes with the caveat 'for his or her age' or, more often: 'He or she must have been beautiful . . . handsome . . . when younger.'

Take Alan Franks interviewing Diana Rigg, in her mid-fifties, in *The Times* telling us how he used to drool over her as a young lovely, and acknowledging that she is still highly desirable but then it comes: 'I . . . have to confirm that she looks remarkable for fifty-five.'

There is probably nowhere on earth where fear at the visible onset of ageing is greater than in Hollywood. Joan Goodman, a journalist with an astute grasp on the price of life in Tinsel Town, who has spent many years interviewing stars and writing about them, explains: 'Insecurity in this place is rampant and it is almost impossible to find anyone who tells their true age. I know men of thirty-five in Hollywood who have collagen injected into their cheeks, right close to their eyes, so they won't get wrinkles and if I ask, "Aren't you afraid of having that done?" they say "I'm more afraid of not having it done." A very successful British actor in his fifties has had lipo-suction on his back because he's lived too well and put on weight and he looks like an old man. At the age of twenty performers are already beginning to save for plastic surgery, as you and I might save for a mortgage.

'You can imagine the mental effect of knowing that a natural process you are going through is going to be the figurative death of you. That devastates people and they just collapse. They see themselves as worthless vessels.'

Actress Suzie Stone lives on the outskirts of Los Angeles and in recent years has been looking to supplement her acting with journalism. She is forty-eight, a tall, shapely, frankly gorgeous woman who believes that being black but light skinned and European in features has enabled her to create an individual niche that has helped make the age problem less pressing. She says: 'I'm not one of a zillion tanned blondes who look so alike they could come off a production line, so the youngest looking ones who can halfway act get chosen. Women here – even those in their sixties and seventies – tend to make up the way they did when they were at their peak even if that was when they were twenty. They wear girlish fashions and long hair in a desperate attempt to look like the younger version of themselves but of course the real-life younger version is there to replace them.

'I don't fit a category, and particularly for promotional work which involves selling a fantasy, I am seen to be glamorous and I can be a little sharp and funny or witty. That's allowed from me and it makes my age more acceptable. But for all that I am very aware that I will get less and less opportunities as the years go on. So many people here just say: "I'm not working. I'm over. I'm finished."'

This sounds familiar to Dudley Moore who has made his home in Los Angeles and well knows how unacceptable it is to be a living demonstration of the inevitability of ageing. Indeed when he asked his agent whether he had other people on his books who might be willing to talk to me for this book he was horrified. Moore tells: 'His reaction was typical – "What is this? Are you going to be featured in some geriatric magazine or something?" I don't think many people are keen on this kind of thing here. It's a society where looks are eulogized over and it does mean people too often give up in despair because they can't take the way they are treated.' He mocks the cruel reality of the world he inhabits: 'I can imagine the conversation with a producer who would like to use me but is worried ... let's use Dudley Moore ... no ... get me a Dudley Moore lookalike ... No get me a young Dudley Moore.'

Nor does the discarding of the ageing person stop in front of the camera. Writer Brian Moore, a charming, weathered man in his sixties, served aromatic tea in the sitting room of his shady wooden house perched high over the bay of Malibu when I visited him there. He shuns meetings, publicity and the glare of exposure.

For him the task is to produce the finely honed prose which has won him several awards and international appreciation and, one suspects, there is in this an awareness of how the fact that he is clearly a man in later life could act against him. He has seen the cruelty of ageism around him: 'There's no tenure for anybody. It helps if you become very famous but ultimately there's no protection. I knew John Huston and when he got old nobody wanted to make a film with him. In this place age is a taboo subject and old people are warehoused so we don't have to look at them.'

The self-hatred engendered by a society with such a value system can be measured in Hollywood through drug and alcohol abuse, the constant breakdown of relationships, widespread depression and pathological fear of being usurped by others.

To find oneself unacceptable, to buy an outside valuation which is based on surface appearance and devoid of any human or spiritual content can be powerfully destructive as was exemplified in the suicide of Marilyn Monroe. For her, I believe, the prospect of ageing, of no longer having the currency of looks which had been the one source of real attention and –

albeit often spurious – love in her life, clearly represented a fate worse than death.

Indeed for years leading up to her actual physical death she seemed to be on a path of psychic suicide. The drugs she took, the unhappiness she could not overcome, showed in her face and body, and she cannot have been unaware that her studios were not amused. What dreadful fear was engendered at the idea that the looks on which not just her career but also her lovableness depended, might be lost. Monroe may be the most memorable, the most popular example of this, but she is certainly not the only one.

Hollywood is instructive as the place where almost everything is exaggerated, distorted, and given a surreal meaning, but finding self-esteem slipping, disgust at what we are becoming as we age, is something people living ordinary lives, light years from Tinsel Town, also experience. Lila Barton, a woman in her mid-forties, much respected in her work as a landscape gardener, and loved by a close circle of friends, regards herself with a kind of loathing as she gets older. This large, voluptuous woman with a mass of steel grey curls and a face full of wit and character says: 'I don't think of the person me, but the body me. I think of myself in terms of other people looking at an ageing, overweight middle-aged woman. I hate myself for thinking it because what does it matter? Why does it matter? The people I'm close to, whom I love and who love me, don't see me in this way. But that doesn't stop what I feel even though I know it's damaging and it's clipping against the wind.'

Michael, in his early forties, fears the repugance he will feel towards his aged face and body, voicing it in the way he talks of others: 'I am almost fanatical about working out. I can't bear to see people who let themselves go as they age. I am convinced that if I look after myself I can remain youthful and when I look around and see what it means to be old that is very definitely what I want. I wonder what it is that changes one into a person who seems to droop, who gets that baggy look around the face and eyes, who may be an awfully nice person but looks – well, past it. It is the thing I fear so much because I know what attitudes are adopted to people like this.'

I have so far looked at the influences on us which colour and manipulate how we may feel about our ageing looks, and these apply to men as well as women. But there are, of course, particular issues for women whose livelihood and acceptability have relied on pleasing men and who have defined themselves according to men's desires. In taking an overview of post-war research, the authors of a paper on images of ageing point to how thoroughly 'women's power is, traditionally, based almost entirely on physical beauty and, unlike the power of men which is built upon more enduring foundations such as wealth and occupation, is bound to fade away.'

I wonder if anyone has expressed more succinctly the efforts men have made, through the exercise of power to make women answerable to their wishes and fantasies, than fashion historian James Laver when he wrote: 'Man in every age has created woman in the image of his own desire.'

There have been changes and feminism has strengthened women in recognizing and opposing male dominance in many areas of life, but for all that women's looks continue to carry a far higher premium in the market place than do men's. So as Rita Freedman observes, mid-life impacts harder on women than men: 'Men do not experience a precipitous drop in social value as they reach mid-life, in the way women do.' She goes on to suggest that it can be particularly hard for the woman who has been beautiful: 'A fading face is experienced as an overwhelming assault to someone whose good looks have always brought her instant attention.' Studies show that those women who were prettiest in college suffer more adjustment problems during middle age.

Yet Barbara Jonson, now fifty-one, is not alone in feeling that she likes her looks better with maturity: 'I was very ordinary looking and rather overweight in my teens and early twenties, so I didn't feel I could dress in trendy clothes or make the most of being young – in fact I was so shy I hid myself away in very nondescript outfits. As I've grown up and had a family and work, I've felt more sure of myself. It means I choose bolder clothes, but I also make sure they really flatter me and aren't just fashionable. I make my face up and I have a smart haircut, and frankly I believe I look better than I did when I was younger.'

Gary, a male nurse in his forties, agrees: 'I was spotty and I was very bony and small looking. I always kept myself out of the spotlight and I lived in blue jeans and T-shirts. I certainly didn't feel admired for my youth. Whereas now I'm a bit stockier, which I like, the spots have gone and I've made my way in the world. I'm actually a bit thin on top and no oil painting, but I do think I know how to dress and have my hair cut to look good, and I've developed decent dress sense since I've grown up!'

But men do not have to grapple with feeling good about themselves in the way women do, argues writer Susan Sontag: 'Men are not subject to the barely concealed revulsion expressed in this culture against the female body except in its smooth, youthful, firm and blemish-free form . . .' It is difficult to argue with this when you come up not just against modern-day culture but the thoughts of poets such as François Villon, who wrote a peculiarly repellent poem describing an aged woman's shrunken breasts and buttocks, shrivelled hands and thighs which are sticks 'speckled over like sausages'.

But it comes still worse from a man who is supposed to be offering a spiritual way forward. Milarepa, a Tibetan Buddhist, when asked if he would like a beautiful woman to become his wife replies:

> At first, the lady is like a heavenly angel;
> The more you look at her, the more you want to gaze.
> Middle-aged she becomes a demon with a corpse's eyes;
> At life's end she becomes an old cow with no teeth.

Even so men are not exempt from the pain of loss and changing identity which the knowledge that they are visibly ageing brings. Body image studies conducted by psychologists Elaine Hatfield and Susan Sprecher in America in the 1980s found that 45 per cent of men to 55 per cent of women were dissatisfied with their appearance and their feelings echoed what we have heard so often from women, that they believed an attractive face to be more important than empathy and the ability to talk about their feelings. Writer Jill Neikerk notes in the American *Psychology Today* magazine that, as men's bodies through film, TV series, men's magazines and female pin-ups, have come to be objectified in the way that has happened to women in the post-war years, so their awareness of an ideal and their own fading from that has become much more of an issue for them.

Added to this is the fact, Neikerk explains, that: 'There is now a subset of women who themselves are attractive, educated and financially secure, who care about every aspect of the way their men look.' What she goes on to explore is how when women hold greater power in the traditionally male domain, then there is an inversion which has them selecting the youngest and fittest men because they are the most appealing.

In the same magazine psychiatrist Michael Pertschuk led a survey on men's feelings about their body image which found that: 'For more than a century the stereotypical male has been depicted as being . . . largely oblivious of his own body.' It is doubtful this was ever true, he said, but concern with body and image was on the increase, impacted upon as it has been for women with: 'ever-improving technology bombarding us with images of beautiful people living the beautiful life'.

The survey found that men with body image disorders are showing up with increasing frequency in psychiatrists' offices and loss of hair came up as an area of heightened concern because: 'Hair is a traditional signal of youth and power, an index of male virility.' David Gilmore, working with the survey team, spoke out on the degree of suffering he now sees in men: 'The male body like the female's has become a punishing crucible, painfully subjected to the tyranny of a cultural ideal.'

It is hardly surprising then that people choose cosmetic surgery as a way of attempting to minimize or even offset the visible proof that they are ageing. It is a choice increasingly being made: the amount spent annually on cosmetic surgery in the US runs to more than $300 million and, according to medical sociologist Kathy Davis, more than 2 million Americans chose some kind of cosmetic surgery in 1988. The numbers are rising all the time. The percentage of people turning to cosmetic surgery in almost every European country is similar and in the UK the number has doubled in the past decade. The figures include a steadily growing number of men.

So is this the Hollywood syndrome taking over? Are we seeing more and more people in ordinary life sharing what seems to be a pathological fear of the ageing process? I have seen little to suggest so, although often the desire for cosmetic surgery is a wish to attempt to moderate the look of ageing. But whereas in Hollywood people know their tenure in that world probably depends on not being seen to age, in less extreme situations, we may recognize that it is a disadvantage to appear to be ageing. There are certainly people who believe that they are less likely to be disadvantaged at work if they can appear not to be ageing too fast, and others feel they can hold on to an identity they value if they choose cosmetic treatment. The fashionable approach in many of the clinics in Europe is for what Vivian Forsyth, who works as a manager in a big company and had a face-lift in her late forties, describes as 'maintenance' – a way of trying to slow down the dropping, sagging and wrinkling of skin, or to pull a body which has spilled its original boundaries too far over passing years, into a trimmer form. Marlene Phillip, the wife of a rural priest, talks of her breast implant as 'compensating for having breasts which have shrunk with the menopause'.

In making such a choice we may feel that cosmetic surgery is a practical response to a problem, a way of purchasing a look, a change that will make you feel better, rather as you might buy a new dress. And there are plenty of men who feel as forty-nine-year-old advertising man Dan Jenners does, that it is a sensible way of 'staying ahead of the game in a business which favours the young'. He explains: 'My face was becoming quite jowly and sagging and I felt I was looking distinctly middle-aged. I've seen colleagues becoming more and more twitchy because they felt they weren't "with it" any longer and I didn't want the same happening to me. I had a lift and I feel it's made a difference. It's certainly made me feel more comfortable about my body although I'm not sure how much anyone else notices.'

Jackie Sullivan who runs the Surgical Advisory Service in London describes the increasing number of men as well as women coming to her for face-lifts, eye jobs, collagen injections and glycolic acid face treatments as part of a quest for confidence. She says: 'They want some insurance against ageing too quickly at a time when they feel they need to be able to hold their own, in a world that is not kind about people getting older.' She also sees a considerable number of mid-lifers who have been through some traumatic event, a crisis, and who feel it is marked indelibly on their face. She explains: 'I see people who have been through dreadful divorces, they have had a death in the family, they've lost their job and it's been tough. As they come through they want to get back on their feet but they feel they have aged too fast because of the crisis and they want to, as it were, give themselves back the lost time. The boost it gives people's self-esteem is enormous.'

This is how it was for Vivian Forsyth: 'I was ending my marriage. I felt I looked old and weary and the feeling that I looked this way made me very uncomfortable speaking up for myself at work, or even when I got into discussions with friends. It may sound silly and perhaps I should have been able to overcome this, but I just couldn't find a way.

'When I'd had my face-lift I liked how I looked much better, I felt I looked more alert, more bouncy, and that made such a difference. I now go into meetings and feel able to say what I want, and I make sure I'm listened to. I believe it helps me to be taken more seriously as a woman at a time when women do get disregarded because they appear to be the wrong side of the tracks.'

But for all those who make this choice, even while recognizing that by opting for surgery they may be playing into the hands of ageism, there are plenty of others who are harshly critical of such a choice. You would be hard put to find anyone disapproving of the efforts people make through exercise, taking vitamins, swallowing anti-ageing pills and elixirs or following so-called age-retarding special diets, to remain youthful-looking. Yet those who decide they will aim for this effect via the scalpel may find themselves having to run the gauntlet of severe criticism.

Why? Isn't choosing surgery, or any other treatment to deal with the way we feel in a complex and pressurized world, a purely personal choice? It seems not. And there are two arguments, one the moral and one the frankly paternalistic, even though it is most often espoused from the mouth of feminism.

One argument has it that in choosing cosmetic surgery we act against the greater good of those who do not want to resort to such methods. In other words we should face the world as nature intended because we may otherwise steal a march over others who cannot or will not go the same path. But this is preposterous. The same people who argue this would almost certainly protest our right to individual freedoms as regards how we feed, pamper, dress and adorn our bodies. That, as much as cosmetic surgery gives people an advantage if they can afford the best. Besides, manipulating our appearance is an age-old, culture-wide approach. Psychologist John

Liggett has made a fascinating exploration of the many ways in which people through the ages have attempted to alter their appearances in the interests of beauty. In *The Human Face* he states: 'There is so much diversity in all the physical effects of ageing. The kind of work one does, for example, is an important factor: another is climate. Consequently the outdoor worker tends to keep his fresh, young-looking colour much longer than the sedentary worker. Chronic ill-health often leaves clear marks on the face, as does a life-time of careless diet and self-indulgence. But constitution is all-important; individuals vary a great deal in their response to physiological abuse. Enormous constitutional differences are to be found between individuals of similar age and racial group in both texture and wrinkling of skin and in freshness of colouring.'

So is it less of a failure for the woman or man who ages very quickly and suffers the disadvantage of this situation to choose cosmetic help, than the person who is about average? If a person has been very handsome or beautiful are they more of a failure because their vanity is so clearly the reason they opted for surgery – and little is abhorred like vanity? And so on. And where does the argument go with those like Cindy Jackson who, when her contemporaries were looking young and cute, spent her years 'as a plain, dumpy prematurely middle-aged looking girl. I felt miserable and grew up inhibited about my appearance which had a profound effect on what I felt able to do and experience, I believe,' she says.

Since she inherited a considerable sum of money in her thirties, Cindy, a small-town American, has spent many thousands of dollars and endured operations every year for the past decade, in order to become, in her own words, a human equivalent of the Barbie doll. She has had a nose job, an eye job, her lips implanted and enlarged. There have been tucks and injections to the face, liposuction to stomach and thighs and assorted other bits of tinkering with what nature provided.

She is very clear indeed that she made a choice about empowerment and the right to be the person she wishes. She defies anybody to tell her she was wrong to take advantage of solutions which are part of the age we live in and which, she insists, have given her great satisfaction. She has now set up a cosmetic surgery advisory service.

Adopting a predictable victim-of-oppressive-paternalistic-forces line, journalists write in pitying tones of what Cindy has come to, but she sees it otherwise: 'I like myself better than I did before. I feel I am the person I want to be and I make no secret of the fact that I chose the help that is available to achieve this. Some people may believe they are making an important stand by suffering when it hurts, but I see what I have done as taking charge of my life and making it work for me.'

If we believe that feminism is about supporting women in the choices they make, as I do, then surely we should respect Cindy Jackson and others for this choice. But the second argument takes a different line and one which has been a bedrock of feminism. It is that women for centuries have adorned, distorted and starved their bodies in order to please men in societies where men's approval has frequently dictated the opportunities and standard of living women achieve. This is true, and the process starts young with little girls being taught to beautify themselves, growing into teenagers who see the route to success as dependent on how gorgeous they can become – although my observation is that, in some areas of society at least, that is changing as, with increased education girls become more sure of their intellect and abilities.

The twenty-something Naomi Wolff wrote an impassioned volume, *The Beauty Myth*, exposing her own discovery of the powerful beauty culture in which she had grown up. And although some older feminists criticized her for writing as though she had discovered something new on a subject which had been much written about in the earlier days of modern feminism, it seems to me a thoroughly good thing that a new generation of feminists should see political issues their own way and express them in their own words. It also seems likely that Wolff's own peers will listen to her and identify with her.

But when the argument is applied to middle-aged women or men, whether they are choosing cosmetics or cosmetic surgery, at a stage in life when, in other ways they are credited with having matured enough to make their own decisions, I see it differently. It may be beneficial to us to understand the under-lying forces which work to persuade us that we want to look younger, as I have already discussed, and understanding these may lead us either to deal better with the ageing process or to make different decisions about how we deal with it, but the decision we make should not bring condemnation for our failings.

Germaine Greer writes: 'The woman who does not wish to dump or deny a part of herself will not try to junk her used face,' while Susan Faludi, another young woman, surveying, quite correctly, a backlash against feminism, takes the line that women are blindly and lemming-like, seeking out cosmetic beauty solutions which do them harm: 'Following the orders of the 1980s beauty doctors made many women literally ill. Antiwrinkle treatments exposed them to carcinogens. Acid face peels burned their skin. Silicone injections left painful deformities. And the beauty industry helped to deepen the psychic isolation that so many women felt in the 1980s by reinforcing the representation of women's problems as purely personal ills.'

Yet is this true? Feminist Rita Freedman has explored the beauty industry and sees a far more complex situation: 'The face-lift has been described as a mid-life passage that leads regressively backward rather than progressively forward . . . but more and more women are choosing this rite of passge because it is so rewarding. The face-lift is being sought by many psychologically healthy females who take an active problem-solving approach to life; by career women who decide they need it for professional life; by single women who feel they need it for social survival.

'These women want to get rid of their self-conscious preoccupation with a cosmetic distraction in order to turn their attention to more important things.'

Freedman acknowledges that an ageist society may force women (and presumably men too) into this 'solution' and that with the pressures there are around remaining youthful, some people look for far more than cosmetic surgery can deliver: 'Those who expect the surgeon to deliver a new mate, anchor a wandering one, or fashion a radical new lifestyle are disappointed ... but the vast majority of face-lift patients feel pleased with the results.' She concludes that: 'Women who seek a surgical solution to the double standard of ageing may be making a healthier response than those who withdraw into a depressive state.'

Medical sociologist Kathy Davis, who conducted a survey of women choosing cosmetic surgery and reported on it in *Reshaping the Female Body*, also from a feminist perspective, found that a good many women are choosing cosmetic surgery because they believe it helps them to maintain an identity they value. They talk of being more sure of themselves and therefore more able to be authoritative after their surgery.

She acknowledges that they might not feel this way in a society that had a different value system for women or the ageing people, but given that these are the realities they are grappling with she came to empathize with their reasoning. She started out on her study with the belief that women are coerced into the choice they make by an oppressive culture which seeks to control and 'normalize' women through their bodies. So when she first learned that a feminist friend was going for breast enlargement because she could no longer stand being flat-chested, Davis was startled at how shocked she was and how difficult she found it to 'hear' her friend's reasoning. It was this which determined her to gain a deeper understanding of the type of women seeking cosmetic surgery and their motivations.

Through the process of carrying out three empirical studies

which involved interviewing women and following them through their operations and the aftermath, she came to understand that these women made the choice after considerable thought and analysis. They regarded cosmetic surgery as something morally problematic which had to be justified, and which aroused contradictory feelings, but they nevertheless felt they were making a legitimate choice and were clear about their reasons and their right to make the decision.

Davis explains: 'For a woman who feels trapped in a body which does not fit her sense of who she is, cosmetic surgery becomes a way to renegotiate her identity through her body.' Rather than cosmetic surgery being submissive, Davis came to see it as enabling women to exercise power in a society based on conditions 'not of their own making'.

This was certainly the way Molly Parkin, now in her sixties, describes it. She wrote vividly in *A Certain Age* of turning to cosmetic surgery having first let her hair grow grey, her face assume its natural wrinkles with falling flesh, until one day she came face to face with her reflection in the mirror and realized she no longer recognized herself. She recalls: 'I went for a face-lift. I had the whole works – eyes, chin, everything – and I felt restored to myself. I had grown sick of so many people asking me if I was exhausted because I looked it, or unhappy because I appeared so miserable. I was thrilled with my face-lift and would recommend one to anybody who like me wants to appear as radiant on the surface as she feels inside.'

In writing in this way, and at length, about cosmetic surgery, I am not setting out to provide an apologia for it, nor to argue that it is something people should be encouraged to choose. It may indeed be honourable, and ultimately a greater source of inner contentment and satisfaction for those who want to deal this way with a culture which is so appalled at the sight of the ageing face and body. And there are wonderful role models such as Georgia O'Keeffe and Bertrand Russell, to name just two well-known people who aged with a great many wrinkles and other clear indications that they were elders, but who were seen as looking good nevertheless. And undoubtedly it is those who go this natural path who will take the lead in doing as Freedman hopes and 'reconstruct an image of ageing that will permit those who have wrinkled in the face of time to look more sympathetically at the map etched on their skin.' So that: 'We trace with pleasure rather than erase with fear the lifelines of experience, allowing our bodies to tell the truth about where we have been.'

Certainly those of us who feel enough affection for ourselves, who feel strong and proud of who we are, may choose to do this and celebrate doing so as Germaine Greer does. But not everybody wishes or feels able to go that path and my point is that those who do not and who choose intervention should not be made to feel that they are frail of character, traitors to the cause, oppressed victims or have to be susceptible to abuse by those who choose not to have it.

The way we dress does not interfere with the natural process of ageing and so you might think that the way we dress would be a matter for ourselves and our individual tastes. After all dress is about expressing who we are and can be one of the most effective ways of feeling good about ourselves. So one of the benefits of ageing should be that we feel free to break 'fashion' rules, be eccentric, colourful, playful, careless or to use all the knowledge we have gleaned through the years to achieve a chic that would have been impossible in younger years.

Instead, all too often people reach mid-life and it is as though they feel they should make themselves as inconspicuous as possible, discreet as can be in subdued clothes and unremark-able hairdos. People who have dressed flamboyantly and with a delightful sense of the anarchic, talk of feeling they have to grow up, not make a fool of themselves, beware of the mutton-dressed-as-lamb criticism and so on.

I know it is precisely how I found myself behaving. My moment of reckoning came in the form of sheeny, velvet leopardskin leggings. There they hung on the market stall among the black and grey lycra leggings, bold and sassy, the stuff of jejune exhibitionism. For half an hour I hovered around the stall, coming back, gazing covertly then averting my eyes when the spider-limbed fashion victim in charge looked in my direction. I had been wearing leopardskin leggings since my early thirties and had always seen them as a kind of jaunty trademark, a touch of outré flamboyance permitted to a thirty-something mother juggling kids and freelance work. During my forties leopardskin tights came into fashion so that seemed to make it all right to replace my well-worn pairs.

But now I was about to turn fifty and I realized that these tantalizing tights embodied all the dark lurking fears and uncertainties which had begun to amass during my forties and which I had somehow pushed away as I protested loudly how absolutely fine it would be becoming fifty. It was almost as though a switch had been thrown and I was pitched into hellish turmoil, a barrage of questions about what being fifty means was unleashed. What prohibitions slide into place as you pass this threshold? If I bought the leggings would I be praised for the determination to go on being the same old me or what kind of clownish outlaw might I become?

Conviction faltered and died. I turned my back on those leopardskin leggings and walked. It was an act of defeatism and I knew it. Call it giving in gracefully, a dignified recognition of the need to find a new way of being, but to me it felt like a full-stop writ large at a point in my life when I didn't want it there.

Such thinking, I believe, needs kicking out of court very fast. It is a tyranny of the worst kind and, as I shall discuss later, here too we are prone to hidden persuaders. I was shocked at the level of prescriptiveness and proscriptiveness which greets us as we reach the middle years. The pleasure that is taken in youthful experiment, sartorial anarchy and inventiveness, the freedom of the young to dress as they wish is transformed into a dreadful, dreary puritanism for the middle-aged person. We are told loud and clear and publicly, in no uncertain terms what is and is not acceptable as dress and style once you attain that hideous euphemism, 'a certain age'. Writer Alison Lurie observes: 'Deviation from the sartorial code . . . tends to meet with a largely critical response.' Indeed.

Consider this attack on a talented, good-looking, middle-aged woman, long salivated over by reporters as sexual dynamite, who chooses in her late forties, to display herself as she wishes: 'Yesterday's picture of actress Helen Mirren was a lesson in how not to dress when you have reached a certain age . . . transparent chiffon does no favours to anyone who no longer has the taut diaphragm and slender waist of youth.'

While Goldie Hawn was designated winner of the *Daily Mail* annual Mutton Dressed as Lamb Award after she was photographed from the back wearing a see-through dress in which she revealed a sliver of flesh around the top of her waistband. She was ticked off for not realizing she has become one of those 'women who, despite reaching a certain age, still insist on wearing dresses that reveal where they should conceal . . . women who haven't yet realized their figures are past their sell-by date.' The press, which has eulogized to the point of idiocy over Hawn's pouting, tousle-haired girlish charms, cannot tolerate those charms in a more mature form, or the fact that she feels good about showing them.

Nor is the middle-aged man exempt from this kind of judgmental assault. The *Daily Mail* deemed 'mutton dressed as ram' those who reveal bodies that are less than galvanized steel in clothes decreed as suitable for younger men. Writer Anne de Courcy opined: 'Men are even worse [than women]. Too-tight jeans belted in under a beer belly, shirt buttons popping to give an impromptu view of an unpleasantly convex torso, the long hair of careless youth hanging beneath the bald dome of twenty years later.'

Quite why it should look foolish to continue wearing clothes we have enjoyed and which we have felt reflected our personalities through earlier years is a question we should ask ourselves.

But we are told in myriad articles, opinion columns, television and radio talks, as well as implicitly through who is photographed or filmed wearing certain styles of dress, and who is not, what is and is not acceptable. I have already said that I have been shocked at what a storm of unwritten legislation is pumped at us about how we should deal with the business of our appearance at mid-life. What comes through very clearly is that carrying on as we have done will not do. Anna Wintour, editor of American *Vogue*, is just one of a posse of women and men in the fashion world whose aesthetic senses are shaped by this obsessive world and whose words, brought to us through the media, have disproportionate authority. Like anxious rats in Armani jackets they twitch and sniff looking for some aberration to criticize, some fragile self-esteem to shoot down because its owner has offended against their self-styled sartorial code. Wintour states: 'Nothing is sadder or more frightening than seeing a woman of the more interesting age in clothes too girlish or revealing. It makes her appear as if she is out of touch with herself. And she is.' Really? Perhaps she enjoys those clothes, feels her body looks good in them, prefers the feel and effect of them to structured jackets and well cut shirts. I can point to plenty of middle-aged women, and men, who wear what are deemed youth clothes and look sensational because they have developed unique style and they feel good the way they are. The fact that they have wrinkles on the face, and hands beginning to go the way of crepe paper, in no way diminishes how good they look.

Do we unquestioningly accept it when Lesley Cunliffe writing for British *Vogue* relegates those who cannot or do not wish to abide by her idea of style to the realms of insanity: 'To cling pathetically to the style of one's youth is a sign of dementia.' Men who do not wish to sober up as they grow up also come in for a good deal of attack. Mick Jagger photographed at fifty in what I would call a dazzling reassurance that half a century need not consign men to the man-made fibre slacks and chain-store woollies – velvet waistcoat, satin shirt and jeans on a beautifully maintained body – was ticked off in a range of publications from the austere *Guardian* to the tabloids for being stuck in a time warp. While Rosalind Miles quotes a criticism of Bill Wyman as an ageing idol 'prancing around in clothes which look ridiculous on men twenty years younger, trying to live up to some pathetic image he thinks he has to maintain.'

Negotiating the mid-life years is daunting enough and what we need is to be praised for boldness, inventiveness, a refusal to give up on wearing certain clothes, styling our hair, painting our faces in ways which feel good and connect us to the libido. What we do not need is articles instructing us that long hair is inappropriate for over forties, that we should tone down the colours we wear, settle for sensible low-heeled pumps. It prompted Madeline Moseley, who dares not trust her own instincts and judgment, even though she knows her body and her personality more intimately than anyone, to write to the *Guardian*: 'When will I be too old to wear jeans any more? Do I already look ridiculous in them? . . . I've got some grey hair now, though my blonde hair conceals it nicely, or so I tell myself. Are people already eyeing me in jeans and plaid flannel shirts and saying "How sad" or "How absurd"?' More absurd, I think, is the fear we feel of disapproval if we put on jeans if we feel like it.

Reflecting on all this it seems to me vital that, if we do not wish to tone down, fade down or take on a kind of tailored chic which is deemed appropriate, we make a very visible protest. I can't help feeling that we would do better to take Jenny Joseph as guru, with her wonderful inspirational poem 'Warning' than to be terrorized by fashion arbiters:

> When I am an old woman I shall wear purple
> With a red hat which doesn't go, and doesn't suit me.
> And I shall spend my pension on brandy and summer gloves
> And satin sandals . . .'

Certainly this is the view of Maggie Clarke, sixty-four, a

Devon farmer whose face and body tell of years spent labouring in the outdoors, but who refuses to apologize for this by wearing 'appropriate' clothes. She is to be found in flouncy gipsy skirts with tops tied under the bust, tight leggings and Top Shop T-shirts in boiled-sweet colours. Her long dark hair is, more often than not, worn hippie style and hanging to her shoulders. Mavis Hoyle, fifty-three, delights in her, 'long red nails, bleached hair and bright colours' and says, 'I don't mind if people think I'm odd. I don't at all believe in growing old gracefully.'

Or there is the jauntiness of Bob Wood who says: 'I feel good in jeans and loud T-shirts and sneakers, and I even wear a baseball cap sometimes. Do I look like someone trying to be sixteen? Do I care? If others don't like it they can look away. It's their problem not mine.'

Writer Alice Thomas Ellis who, at sixty, has a gently creased face capped with a turban scarf, her body hidden in the folds of a long loose dress, says that making mid-life an expression of who we are and feeling good with it means: 'seeing the pleasure in becoming something different while hanging on to our authenticity.'

But authenticity, as I see it, is about holding on to who and what we feel ourselves to be and isn't that what Mirren and Hawn were doing? By wearing the clothes they chose and thus exposing themselves, I believe they bravely confronted and even mocked the inhibition and anxiety which exists around older people's sexuality, the fear that it is somehow aberrant and inappropriate. Isn't it possible that those writers and editors who passed public judgment on these two women are full of conflict about their own ageing bodies and fearful of their fading desirability? Highly probable I would say. For it is fear that makes us reach for the chain-store separates that Rose, a West Indian whose sartorial bravado in mid-life is a delight, describes as 'dresses like envelopes'; it is fear which fits out a myriad of men in the style-challenged grey suit, a kind of middle-age purdah.

In the ageing body we see disintegration and that is unbearable. Why else would there be such fear and loathing expressed
at the sight of 'inappropriate' dressing? Is the woman who
insists on sporting Top Shop gear when she is sixty really such
an offence to our eyes and sensibilities that she deserves
retribution through the press, an attack *de haut en bas* from
the fashion arbiters? What harm does it do unless it is so
unsettling that it sparks our own internal fears?

Those fears are so much the greater because we do not
know how to present ourselves, to negotiate our changing
appearance, to feel conviction in who we are. If, instead of
coming up against hostility for the choices we make about our
mid-life physical beings, we were given support, it might do
much to temper the already conflicting and complex feelings
many people experience at this time.

There are signs that things are shifting and we should not
rule them out of court because they tend to happen in the
world of showbiz, for public personalities are valuable as
groundbreakers, icons of possibility. Joan Collins, Tina
Turner, Cher may not be what you or I want to be, or could
be, but they have made the point that it is possible to be
something other than invisible and asexual at mid-life and it
was remarkable how many women and men I interviewed
chose them as role models.

Glamour and femininity when it is construed as moulding
and creating the female being to suit man's design and desire,
is a difficult area. As discussed in the context of cosmetic
surgery, women who have battled for equality and recognition
quite understandably do not applaud others who demonstrate
what is read as obeisance to male power in the way they
present themselves. Yet there is a considerable difference, it
seems to me, between the young, unformed, insecure girl
searching to create an identity, who pins her colours to the flag
woven with threads from a patriarchal value system, and the
woman at mid-life who has decided that glamour is the style,
the approach, the way of celebrating her body, that appeals.

I would argue that glamour and the raunchy sexuality it embodies is something which can only be achieved with a maturity that embodies a confident libido, good feelings about oneself, a degree of self-parody and certainly awareness of the game being played. I do not see it as the posturing of a pathetic mid-lifer who is trying to offset the knowledge of ageing, so much as the bold statement of a woman who feels she is entitled to the grand display.

Racquel Welch has certainly pursued the cult of glamour and, as feminist academic Camille Paglia points out, in doing this she has carved a niche, a status indeed, which would have been most unlikely if she had stormed Hollywood in dungarees and house-mouse style. Paglia, in what may well be regarded as a maverick gesture, designated Racquel Welch as THE role model for women in the 1990s, when she interviewed her for *Tatler* magazine, an accolade which not only celebrates Welch's enjoyment of her sensuality, sexuality, and femininity, but makes the point that it has matured and developed to become something far more powerful so that now, as a woman in her fifties, Welch has a strength and confidence which informs the way she has styled herself.

Her overtly glamorous and sexual looks are not the desperate striving of a pubescent kid to fit male fantasy, but the calculated persona of a woman who runs her own life, I would argue. While Paglia's line is that: 'Racquel parallels the whole sorry saga of what has gone wrong in the last twenty-five years in the Anglo-American women's movement. Her public presence is simultaneous with a powerful movement for reform within feminism, which must recover its sexuality. In her quest for self-determination and for harmony of mind and body, Racquel is an ideal role model for women of the Nineties.'

Certainly I would agree that she is one outstanding role model. The important point about being a generation of mid-lifers forging new ideas around the appearance of ageing, is that we should have a galaxy of role models representing different looks, lifestyles, value systems. It should be whatever it is we want it to be and care to present to the world. It is the variety of looks and the confidence of those displaying them which will challenge ageism more effectively than prescriptive rules on what is appropriate and politically correct.

The irony in all the angst about the ageing appearance is that it disregards how little confidence the young often have in *their* appearance. They may be admired and envied by their elders but often, as so many of us remember, it is a time of seething insecurity about the way you are and how to style yourself. And it is certainly true that some people genuinely do prefer the way they look as they age. Hilda, now forty-six and running a bar with her husband tells of being a 'distinctly plain and rather shrunken creature' when young. She laughs at the memory as she says: 'I hated the way I looked then but now I can look in the mirror and say, hand on heart "you look pretty good, old girl". It's not that I'm a beauty, just that my body has filled out a bit and I like that. I've found a hairstyle that works and I have several dress styles from very casual to ultra smart which make me feel good because I think I've learned through the years to pick the things that actually work on me.'

Forty-three-year-old David, who works for BT, wore fashionable straight-leg jeans, a white T-shirt, pistachio green linen jacket and trainers when we met. He remembers a childhood where there was little money for clothes and he often had second-hand things. 'I never felt good about myself, and in my teens I was terribly shy because I saw myself as much less attractive than other boys. I never wore anything flash, even when I got into my twenties and could afford it. But I've become more confident as I've got on in the world and I remember quite clearly one day going into a shop to try on some trousers because I needed them. Instead of taking the most basic and inoffensive I took a pair with pockets and stitching, and in slightly shiny fabric. I also took a very loud shirt. They sound awful now but they were really an important step for me. I bought them and then I went and had a new haircut, sort of brushed forward instead of slicked back as I had had it. I really liked the way I looked and I suppose because of this other people commented on how good I looked. I went on from there to develop quite a strong style and these days I thoroughly enjoy clothes and I wear quite a lot of stuff you find in the boutiques aimed at younger men. But I think it's all about confidence and that's what I've got in middle-age.'

David and Hilda are fortunate in having developed the confidence to feel they look better at mid-life than they did when younger. Others may be helped to see the possibility that mid-life can be a time when fashionable and even daring clothes can look good on the catwalk. This is one of the most public places where we see mid-lifers standing proud as examples of fashionable looks, albeit on a small scale so far, on the catwalks of famous fashion designers. Brenda Polan, who now works as fashion director for *YOU* magazine and is former fashion editor of the *Guardian* talks of how Japanese designers like Comme des Garçons and Issey Miyake regularly use older models; Pat Cleveland now in her forties is to be seen, and Twiggy who almost invented the cult for models who look like your youngest daughter, looked at least as beautiful as when she was young in a recent high-gloss fashion spread. Increasingly, too, older men feature in fashion shows and in the pages of magazines in which they model stylish clothes. One of the most beautiful examples, to my mind, was an advertisement for Banana Republic clothes in which a man and a woman, probably in their seventies were used to model casual clothes.

Yet while such models are inspirational they seem remote from us more ordinary mortals. By contrast a fashion-spread in the *Independent on Sunday* which featured a range of people of different types, colour, and class, from fifty upwards, wearing clothes they visibly enjoyed, was the best inspiration imaginable, and wouldn't it be encouraging if more magazines – and particularly the fashion heavy glossies – would follow this idea?

So far I have discussed attitudes around the ageing appearance and how we may galvanize the courage to do as we wish with our mature looks. But then no less important may be finding a new way of valuing our looks as we age. When Judith Paige went into menopause in her late forties she felt dispirited, unsure of herself and had a sense of life drawing in as her children prepared to leave home. It was her daughters who spotted her potential and urged her to try for some modelling work. Rather hesitantly she took a weekend modelling course and afterwards she was asked to do a photo session and be on the agency's books. She could not believe the results and says, laughingly: 'The photos had to be of someone else. I looked good, I was not as smooth-skinned and fresh-faced as I had assumed but still . . .'

She laughs still more recalling how, a few months and a couple of low-key jobs later, she was photographed naked from the waist up for the cover of *Lears*, a glamorous women's magazine started by editor Frances Lear specifically to create a new image of and for older women. That was followed by an article and photograph in *Advertising Weekly* of Brooke Shields in a similar pose saying: 'Brooke, here's what you're going to look like in thirty years.' Paige was excited and delighted by the way her life had turned, how the menopause, far from being the time she faded from view, has been a time of growth and confidence. She went on to write *The Choice Years*, a book of inspiration and guidance for mid-life women and she says: 'The irony of earning a living with my looks when my looks were supposedly fading at the same rate as my estrogen levels was not lost on me.'

It may be that turning life in a less visible direction brings a new and inspiring look to middle-age. I interviewed Audrey Hepburn a while after she had started working for UNICEF (the United Nations Children's Fund) and had just been to Ethiopia looking at work being done with desperate and hungry children. The face I remembered as beautiful but always with a controlled, taut look, had softened and relaxed.

Her excitement talking about the projects she had seen which really were improving the life of children, the unguardedness of her speech and expressions, brought something quite lovely, soft and warm into her face.

Terence Stamp too, the unbearably handsome, but icily cool young actor has assumed a much softer gravitas, that seems to reflect a calmer more fulfilled life, now that he does little acting, writes, reads a great deal and has turned to spiritual pursuits. He says it himself: 'Being an ageing beauty doesn't worry me. During the 1960s I had come across women like the actress Sylvana Magnana and my yoga teacher, the Countess Wanda, whose physical beauty was being reinforced by a kind of inner dimension and it was a revelation to me. Countess Wanda is eighty-five . . . when you meet her you start thinking about beauty in another way . . .'

Something close to this is, it seems, found in Western countries where ageing continues to be seen to have a value, even while the loss of youth is acknowledged. It is interesting to question why in France and Italy, for example, where sophisticated advertising and a delight in youth are part of the culture, attitudes appear to be other than ours.

For example in France where the expression *un certain âge* conveys a far greater sense of mysterious glamour than our description, fifty-year-old actress Catherine Deneuve, is widely regarded as a great beauty and clearly they don't believe age has devalued her. She acknowledges this gracefully and says she believes that in her country there is an appreciation of someone who is psychologically mature. So it is, she suggests, that they make films which feature older actors, like *Indochine* in which she starred and which, she says: 'capitalizes on spiritual evolution, experience and, yes, why not say it, on their age'. Equally Jeanne Moreau, in her sixties, the wonderful, sensual star of a British TV production of Alice Thomas Ellis' story 'The Clothes in the Cupboard' is quite simply seen as wonderful and infinitely sensual. In the same way the ageing Alain Delon and before he died Yves

Montand were not seen as less desirable and interesting as they aged, and their parts have reflected it.

Angela Wheeler, an English woman, moved to France when she was twenty-one. Now, aged forty-four, she is marrying a Frenchman almost a decade younger than she is. She believes: 'I would feel very uncomfortable, very much as though I had a toy boy if I lived in Britain or America, but here the older woman has a much greater currency. There is an appreciation of sophistication and chic and those are things which people gain through living, through developing a confidence and style of their own.'

Lindesay Ballieu, also English but living in Paris and working as a translator, says that a French woman and a French man with wrinkles and lines will continue to attract looks and be considered sexually desirable provided they look as though they bother about themselves. The French do not despise age in the way English-speaking Western countries appear to do, she says, 'but they do despise the person who does not make the best of themself.'

'In the Latin countries appreciation of older people comes from something different,' according to Paolo Altieri, forty-seven, who works between Britain and Italy. 'Our families are very strong and we gain much knowledge and support from parents and grandparents. I cannot imagine thinking women like my mother were worthless because they do not look like young girls. The other point, talking about women, is that we love women to be mothers, we see that as feminine and sensual and so if they are big and womanly and even a bit worn because of being mothers it is a look that is appreciated. And in the big cities men and women dress in a very elegant way, but often quite sexily and with bright colours. They have a feel for how to do it as they age and I am not alone in thinking that often they look more attractive than younger people.'

It is also so true as to perhaps seem a cliché that people who are engrossed in creativity, passion, political fervour, an intellectual or spiritual journey appear to mind considerably less about the way they look as they get older, than do many others. This is clearly true of artists such as artist Georgia O'Keeffe whose unadorned face was proud and strong; the poet Adrienne Rich whose face is lined and aged, but whose eyes and smile carry the animation of somebody who delights in what she is. Bertrand Russell, fired until the end with his intellectual notions, was creased and lined as a sun-dried prune, but it is the intelligence in his face which is so appealing in the photographs; Yehudi Menuhin's face so well known through pictures, has aged with the years, but it is his quiet composure and then his passion, as he performs, which we observe.

But nobody has illustrated the beauty which exists in contentment with oneself, more powerfully for me, than Ani Lodrho, a Chilean Buddhist monk, now in her sixties. She sits in the fading light of day, perched on the windowsill of the red-brick house she shares with others involved in Tibetan Buddhist teaching and learning, talking with delighted animation about the life she has chosen which has put her outside the normal framework of seeing and being seen, judging and being judged on appearance. Her pale-skinned face with its many lines beneath the shaved head, the smile which spreads like morning sun across an African sky, over her face, the eyes so bright and full of humour and pleasure make her quite stunningly beautiful.

Reaching contentment with our physical changes and how they make us look can be done through many routes but it may require a very conscious effort, particularly as we go on getting older. That is the view of Gay Gaer Luce author of *Your Second Life*, a book which grew out of SAGE (Senior Actualization and Growth Explorations), a group she set up in her native America to help older people explore ways of feeling more positive about where they are in life. In a room in a house outside New York a group of women and men in their sixties and seventies were confronting feelings about their appearance. Luce describes:

As we went round the room everyone felt ashamed. Could we learn to accept wrinkles, baggy skin, scars from operations, fat hips and tummies, gnarled toes? Was it true that older bodies were ugly? At meetings over the following year the group looked more and more intimately at their bodies and discussed how they had come to be the way they were. They turned on its head the way we delight in the 'compliment' of being told how young we look, and took some aspect of the ageing body to talk about in complimentary terms, so that in one exercise the gracefulness, strength and sensuality felt in a pair of wrinkled, veined and gnarled hands was praised.

Something similar, but with a younger, mid-life group was organized in Manchester in the north of England, by a group of late mid-lifers with the aim of helping people, entering this stage of life, to know and like their changing physical self. There were a number of consciousness-raising exercises and in one a woman in her early fifties faced a looking glass: 'Mirror mirror on the wall . . . show me the deeply etched laughter lines, the wrinkles and creases won through the exhausting but exhilarating years of rearing children and working hard; the furrows worn into my forehead through work, learning and thinking – those processes which keep us endlessly developing and growing, a skin weathered and toughened by the business of living; grey hair letting the world know I have maturity with all its virtues on my side.'

A smile broad and sweet stretched over the lined face as she stepped back to make way for a man who, too, had many lines, and thinning hair. He grimaced when I asked how he felt about getting older. But he also said, 'I don't like getting older, but I can see there are compensations and I'm determined to be in the process with others learning to feel differently.'

In the end it is only we at the coalface who can change things and there is probably no tougher battle than the one with looks. But it is a battle we see being taken on by today's mid-lifers of every class and type. The number of older people joining gyms, taking exercise classes, running and swimming, partly for health but also as a way of caring for their appearance, grows steadily, and it shows.

It is cheering too to find that, for all the pressure on us to wrap ourselves in discretion once the middle years hit, a good number of mid-lifers are doing precisely the opposite, defiant in the face of anyone who disapproves. They wear short, short skirts on bodies which are as slim, or often slimmer, than in younger years; they wear the brightest of colours, the sexiest of styles, high heels and bags of jewellery if that is what they like. I see bravura and conviction and that is what is needed if we are to put an end to the corrosive proscriptiveness I have described.

But most importantly if we are to bring about a different perception of ourselves as we age, we need the confidence to feel good about who and what we are. This comes, most certainly, from inner feelings of worth. If we value ourselves we stand the best chance of persuading the world outside to do the same – our faces are the mirror for these feelings and we should be applauded for doing it by whatever means we choose because it is, by any route, a difficult task. We must defy the prohibitions and prescriptions of those whose authority is reductive, not life-enhancing, and move on to say, with conviction and pleasure, as May Sarton did on her eightieth birthday: 'I am more myself than ever.' If we can do this we will have given ourselves a gift and achieved something for the generations behind us looking nervously towards the way mid-life looks.

Critical Time

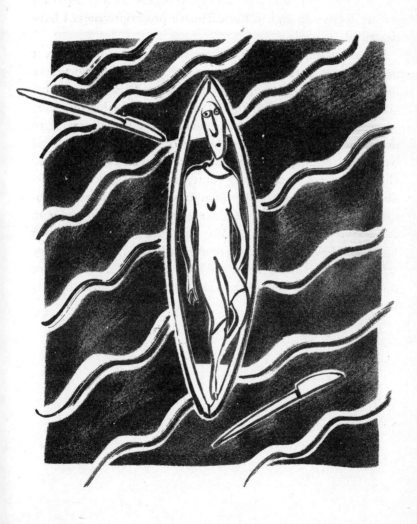

Do I dare
Disturb the universe?
T. S. ELIOT, '*The Love Song of J. Alfred Prufrock*'

THE ACTOR ROBERT STEPHENS was in full dramatic flood describing his mid-life crisis: 'An irresistible force seemed to sweep me up in a kind of madness when I hit forty. I got into a panic, there seemed no way to make sense of my life, I felt everything was over and I had to prove something . . . I wanted to assert myself as a man who was still attractive to women . . . I drowned the fear that perhaps my acting career was finished with booze.'

The words were delivered in a low, carefully pitched voice as Stephens illustrated what he was saying with vast gestures, his long arms and slim tapering fingers thrust outwards while his face mirrored the anguish he was recalling. He sat at the picture window of the flat where he lives with actress Patricia Quinn, watching shadows fall over Primrose Hill in the fading afternoon light. His leonine face was in profile until suddenly he turned and smiled like a big, cheery child who knows there is a happy ending to his story.

I listened to the memories he selected, creating a mosaic of his life, returning over and over to painful memories of a childhood where he could not seem to win his parents' affection or approval and was he says 'a cowering creature, like a dog waiting to be beaten', so that when his mother told him she had tried to abort him when she knew she was pregnant, it made a ghastly kind of sense. Hearing him I was struck by how, even though he has apparently reached some kind of rapprochement with these memories, it was when he reached mid-life that the pain at what had happened in his life appeared to trigger an overwhelming sense of failure and futility. It led him on a path which he now believes was vital. He explained that he now believes he had to go so far down into despair that he feared destroying himself completely, in order to find the conviction to pull his life together again, and it was this which led him, during his sixties, to a stunningly successful renaissance in the theatre. That and a relationship which, he says, finally allows him to trust love.

Stephens described experiencing what he calls his crisis as he moved into his forties, a time when everything was out of kilter and he was unable to draw himself from the self-destruct path. His third marriage, to actress Maggie Smith, had ended and she was living in Canada with their two young sons while he was in Britain. His career had faded out to inconsequential parts – 'a litany of mediocrity' in the words of one critic – and as he 'spiralled ever downwards wrecking all chances I might have had of stabilizing myself, friends drew away because they couldn't get through to me at all . . . I convinced myself I was having a whale of a time and that being forty was fine . . . but underneath it all there was a black terrible sense that nothing was all right at all, the knowledge that I couldn't go on and on fooling myself. And I couldn't. Friends talked of me as becoming louder and rowdier but inside I was howling and desperate. Then my health went down and I almost died. Just before that, in spite of everything, I had got the part of Falstaff in *Henry IV* which was like a dream opportunity at last. Then I collapsed with severe anaemia. When that had been sorted out I forced myself to take stock, to see that I had a choice about whether to waste my life or find a different way of going forward.'

Lesley Barnham, forty-nine, identifies with Stephens' feeling of being caught up in a pattern of behaviour over which there seemed to be no control, and she sees the build-up and her own crisis time as the culmination of growing frustrations, pressures and a depression she had never properly dealt with. As she contemplated getting older and with it a feeling of dark emptiness ahead it was, she says, as though her psyche just went berserk. It was a time during which she watched herself destroy the things she had spent years building up.

She sits in a small rented council house, made pretty by her use of colourful fabrics, the many carefully chosen prints on the walls, the selection of smiling photos of her son George, now at university, at different ages and stages. This is the new, more meagre life she has created for herself since 'negotiating a row with my boss at a large management consultant agency which had head-hunted me for an important well-paid job. I made it impossible to stay. I'm not sure to this day whether I was fired or resigned, but either way it meant that in my mid-forties, as a single mother with huge debts, I was suddenly without a job and unlikely to get freelance work.'

Yet the sense of fear at how she might cope was mingled with 'a colossal sense of relief and release that I had no choice but to change my life'. She is a handsome, well-built woman in leggings, a giant T-shirt and an enormous silk wrap across her shoulders. Her face is relaxed, her mass of steel-grey curls worn loose. The style is laid-back as she describes what happened: 'I was very successful, very young for the work I was doing as a management consultant trainer, and after my husband died when George was very young, I had to earn a living. I enjoyed the work and I felt valued because of what I was paid, but I was very aware of being on a speedtrack all the time. It was high pressure and I had to spend a good deal of time pitching for more work. At home in the evenings the phone rang constantly. George was reaching adolescence and needed time and attention instead of which I was snapping at him, telling him I was too busy or tired for him. I was lonely and depressed because the lover I had was playing around, and it was as though I could feel a head of steam boiling up inside me. There was this growing sense that I might just explode, that things couldn't go on holding together. As you can see I've had to drop my standard of living and there's no security in my life, but I have strength now and faith in myself.'

Both Stephens and Barnham talk of having experienced a mid-life crisis, a phenomenon which is described by those who study human development, as occurring in the middle years. It is judged as different from other crises which may occur in earlier years, because it is seen to be triggered by some event or psychological trauma that has its roots in the fact that we have reached the mid-life stage. Most of us know little or nothing of this and we are unprepared for the often disturbing, unsettling, painful feelings which may occur. Nor can we understand why, in what may appear an utterly random way, we find ourselves questioning just about everything we thought we held dear. We may no longer be able to see the value of all we have striven to achieve in the first half of life. It can seem that everything has gone off course.

The sense described by Robert Stephens and Lesley Barnham of gathering momentum, of an internal chaos which would not be held in check, so that both were forced off course although in very different ways, is echoed by others who have spoken to me or who have poured words onto paper telling how life quite simply would not hold together as it had done for the earlier years, telling of being upended, as though a great wave had swept them off the shore into a sea of doubt, anxiety, self-loathing, contempt for those around and there was a sense that they could no longer bear what they had made of their lives, but had no vision of a better way.

It has been my experience too. During my mid-forties I was filled with a profound discontent at the things I had spent the early years of my life constructing. I was obsessed with the idea that things must change and full of fury at those around for not fulfilling the dreams and ambitions I had for my life. I was so tense you could have played Beethoven's Fifth on my psyche. It seemed that nihilistic invading forces had occupied my mind and there was nothing good about past or future. I too plunged into a dreadful darkness and had to struggle to find a way of living which made me less dependent on external stimuli and approval than I had been for the past forty-five years.

The scary feeling that there is no certain way to make sense of life any more, that the reference points have been blotted and blurred, are common themes. In the words of picture-framer Laurence Hughes, just coming up to fifty: 'I thought there must be something wrong with me that I was feeling so hopeless, that I looked at my four lovely sons and a life which has much good in it, and felt a hollowness about it all. There was nothing dramatic to report. I didn't have a single, serious problem which people would understand. It was just that the feeling of nothing being all right any more had crept over me and wouldn't go away.'

The experiences we perceive as a mid-life crisis are described in myriad ways and they make us feel isolated, lonely because we do not see the same in others, we feel bad, mad and sad at the mutation of emotions, the doubts over what we have spent the years building. We fear going on as we have been doing, and we fear breaking the mould and facing the great open space on our own. It can be a low-level sense of being dislocated from reality, or what Anne Vanderschoot voices as 'not knowing oneself and consequently those nearest to you also not knowing you'. Or what Miranda Mullen, in her early fifties, describes as 'never being sure from day to day how I will feel, whether I will feel love for my partner or an over-whelming desire to leave him; whether the work I do will seem immensely satisfying as it sometimes does, or hollow and pointless; whether I feel myself a mother who has done a good job in loving her children and helping them grow well or whether I throb with guilt at what I fail to do.'

Men talk, again and again, of 'dying inside' and 'suffocating' with the belief that they cannot find a way to experience the intensity and passion they once knew, and are scared rigid at the thought of marching on through many more years with their senses blanked out.

But on the other hand there are people who look askance at the very idea of a mid-life crisis, and those whose lives seem to flow from stage to stage without any outward signs, at least, of the process being problematic. And clearly a mid-life critical time – the way I label the longer-term, more diffused painful feelings as well as the intense cumulative time of a crisis point – is not inevitable. Yet according to a Gallup poll survey (1992) over two-thirds of middle-aged men believe that there is an identifiable phenomenon called the mid-life crisis and over half thought they had either had or were having one at some point around the forty-to-sixty age range.

I have become more and more convinced, while writing this book, that there is some kind of profound questioning, a sense of being isolated with alien, disruptive emotions, feelings of missed opportunities, of an urgent desire to change the texture of life before it is too late, which affects a great number of people. Just how significant both men and women feel their mid-life upheavals to be, was made clear to me time and again. Reactions to my subject matter were fascinating. I would be trapped in corners at parties by people I did not know, unburdening themselves as though grateful to have found an anthropologist who understood their species; there were those who wondered if something was wrong with them because they seemingly had so much and yet felt they had nothing they wanted – they begged me to tell them they were not alone. Others pooh-poohed the whole idea of a mid-life crisis, insisting that was not something they would 'fall for', before telling how they planned to leave a wife and kids in order to discover their spiritual selves; of a compulsion to chuck in a serious career and home they had spent years building up to roar across South America on a motor bike; that they had met someone who spoke to the poetry in their soul and were prepared to leave their children to share a life of poverty with him or her, and so on. These may have been the best things they could possibly have done, I was in no position to judge, but whatever, it seemed there was something troublesome in the state of the human condition.

It is particularly difficult, I believe, for our generations to accept this kind of emotional frailty, coming as it does at a time when we are struggling hard to convince ourselves that things are not changing, that we are going on as ever before, that we still belong to the younger generation. Nor, I believe, are we helped by what seems to be a fashionable tendency in the spate of books and writings coming out on the subject of mid-life, to determinedly paint mid-life as a high-spot in life – if we can just overcome the loss of youth. What we have to celebrate, these peddlers of optimism say, is having reached a stage in life when we may have more confidence and conviction about ourselves than we did when younger, unchained from children we are able to make choices and decisions for ourselves as we wish. It is a time when we can end unsatisfactory relationships, pursue new interests, build plans for a productive future.

All these things can certainly be part of the truth for a substantial number of people – although it is important to remember how thoroughly class, race and social circumstance can affect the picture. But to say that we should feel unambiguous satisfaction at mid-life which is, after all, the time when we begin to face our own mortality, is to undermine those of us who are experiencing difficult feelings about the inevitability of ageing – feelings which can indeed provoke crises, regardless of how much conviction, confidence and pleasure in having more time for ourselves we may also experience.

There are, certainly, good reasons why we may have a better experience of ageing than earlier generations, but there is, I believe, a danger in too simple a picture of the possibility of individual triumph over entropy, so that those who do not feel strong may, by contrast, feel even more alone with their troublesome feelings and fears.

Reluctance to admit to a mid-life crisis is complicated by the fact that it has become something of a cliché and a joke, the subject of pop-psychology articles and jocular books like Christopher Matthew's *The Truth About Life After Forty – How to Survive Middle Age* which invites us to be flip about the whole thing: 'The human race has a great deal to put up with at the

hands of "Dame" Nature . . . it would appear that she enjoys
nothing better than seeing us writhing in shame and agony as
a result of yet another of her practical jokes. The crueller the
trick, the happier she is.' Or there are films like Coline
Serreau's *La Crise*, a tale of a man who loses his wife and
children, his job and his friends one after the other and finds
himself having to learn how to be a new kind of man – the loss
of everything in a Grand Guignol gesture followed by a moral
rehabilitation.

The idea here is that the mid-life crisis is little more than an
affectation, the indulgence of the now maturing ME generations who, fearing that their important place at centre stage is
slipping from grasp, must find a way of getting the focus back
on them. And that seems to be par for the course. There is a
great tendency in most developed Western states to deny
psychological pain, to separate ourselves from those who experience it, in order to show that we have our hands firmly on
life's steering wheel. But I consider it no surprise that just this
button-down and belt-up mentality is widely attributed, by
those who pick up the pieces of these tough talkers when they
fall apart, to the fact that they have not been able to find an
outlet for their pressure-cooker feelings.

I am convinced that it is important for our psychological
welfare and our emotional well-being that we do understand
how genuine the feelings we have, and what we experience as
critical times, may be. Through doing this we may then
be able to recognize the very real psychological gains which
can come from coping with the upheavals of this time –
something that will be dealt with more fully in the following
chapter – and which help us to move forward constructively.

If we refuse to accept that what feels serious should be
taken seriously, but seek to joke it off and distance ourselves
from the experience, suggesting implicitly that it is the weaker,
less balanced mortals who suffer mid-life turmoil, we may also
cheat ourselves. There is a solid body of developmental work
which suggests that, whether you call it a mid-life crisis or

something entirely different, a transitional period is essential if we are to carve something valuable and rewarding out of our growing process. Rather than trying frantically, facetiously, to pretend it's of no consequence or a bit of a laugh, we'd do better to acknowledge that we are faced with the challenge of negotiating the next step forward in life.

We may recognize that things are out of sync', we may be grappling with despair and full of fear that we cannot cope, but how do those who are asked to help deal with what is going on, identify the mid-life crisis? Is there a difference between the mid-life crisis and clinical depression or nervous breakdown?

Consultant psychiatrist Dr Anthony Fry, author of *Safe Space*, a philosophical book in which he explores the ways we may find a place – either an actual physical space or a psychic space within our own being – where we can be quiet, reflective, and grow to feel strong and safe in ourselves, suggests we may look at the mid-life crisis as a condition which has layers. The first may be a crisis of the individual's personal value system – we may find ourselves doubting or even dramatically turning our back on those things we have believed in and seen as the roots of our authenticity, the belief system which has supported us so far through adult life. When this happens, Dr Fry says, we may, rather than face the fear engendered by what is happening, instead become hostile and confrontational towards the people close to ourselves. Then comes psychological distress so that we are aware of feeling bad and of not knowing how to cope or how to get ourselves back to what we regard as our normal selves. Dr Fry sees the first stage of the crisis – when our convictions are on shifting sands but we are not facing up to this – as an impasse. If we cannot find a way to cope with our feelings and our psychological state it is possible that the crisis might turn into a psychiatric state which could be clinical depression or a nervous breakdown. This is the most severe development, however, and not the outcome of the majority of critical times even though some help may be valuable.

Dr Fry explains that whether we react to critical times or a crisis point in such a way that our personal pain becomes a pathological condition depends on the personality of the individual. It may be a question of whether we have support systems and internal resources which give us the strength to hold together. He says:

The feelings which cause one person to become totally dysfunctional, to go into collapse, will cause another pain, stress, a host of anguishing questions, but not necessarily disintegration.

The mid-life crisis is a point at which things stop working and it very often appears as a profound crisis of faith. But the individual reactions to the feelings will be very different. One person will take an axe and smash up the desk in their office, another will slip into deep depression and swallow pills, others become so anxious and tense they don't know what to do or how to move. There are people who will try to blot it all out snorting coke.

Psychotherapist David Smallacombe sees the mid-life crisis as 'throwing people out of kilter temporarily', but often the alien feelings do not appear to have a specific focus, which of course can be very confusing. Ben Timms, a social worker found himself wishing, two years ago at the age of forty-eight, that he could just pack his bags and leave his home, partner and two children, even though there wasn't another woman or an offer of a more enticing lifestyle ahead. He says: 'I know when I felt that I was grovelling in the bottom of a black pit of despair with no knowledge of how to get out, I could look at a life which was holding together as it had done for years, and wonder what on earth this was all about. The fact that it didn't make sense was scary.'

Hilary MacDonald, a fifty-four-year-old nurse was appalled to find an equable happy disposition 'do a somersault' for no apparent reason. She tells: 'I had a job I loved, I had security – a house of my own, a good wage, and lots of friends, and then just like that my whole spirit went down. I can pin the day – I'd been out to the country to visit an old school friend who had a couple of really smashing kids and we'd had lots of fun.

I got home that evening and instead of feeling pleasure and a kind of relief at being in my own place, as I usually did, I remember feeling this intense sense of loneliness. My life just looked so empty and pointless. The feeling was there the next day and the next and it just stayed. I found myself suddenly bursting into tears when I saw friends and I even found my sense of commitment to work was gone. I really felt in despair and I just didn't know what had happened.'

Such feelings may, as we shall see later, be a subconscious assessment of where we have reached in life, and opportunities passed, a sudden recognition of *temps perdu*. Hilary later went into counselling and found herself talking and talking about the fact that she had never had a child, even though, she says: 'I told people over and over that it was just as well I hadn't become a mother because I never really wanted children, and that's what I thought myself.'

When these painful feelings move on to precipitate the literal breakdown of function which becomes what we call a nervous breakdown, it is usually in response to a trigger of the kind already described. Psychoanalyst Peter Hildebrand observes:

This is also a time when conflicts can no longer be dealt with so easily by fight-flight mechanisms. Instead of being able to pick up and go off to another city or country; instead of being able to change jobs or career paths; instead of being able to find another partner, men and women at this age are struggling with the successes of structures and relationships which they have constructed over perhaps one or two decades. Anxiety and depression now come to the fore, as do the psychosomatic manifestations with which we are all familiar.

Understandably we also want to know how to spot a mid-life critical time, or a crisis brewing up, and although there are clear analyses of why they occur – which we will move on to – identifying what may be the beginning of something that will turn into a profound upheaval or will lead you in a direction you cannot at the outset anticipate, may be difficult. One of the difficulties is that critical times do not necessarily occur as a single intense event, but may be a series of smaller eruptions over a period of time and they can take very different forms. We may find ourselves caught in the psychic equivalent of a Wall Street collapse, a sense of the gathering momentum of internal chaos which will not be held in check. But equally the signs can be as quiet as an internal voice softly but insistently demanding to be heard. It may be as psychotherapist David Smallacombe, who hears so many manifestations of the mid-life critical time, in his consulting room, suggests, 'an emotional grumbling appendix'.

Alix Kates Shulman's *Drinking the Rain* expresses how we may be feeling:

As the world grew unfamiliar I began to lose my bearings ... The facts were, my children were suddenly grown and gone; my husband, their father, who worked in a distant city, was increasingly estranged from me; my parents, though still vigorous in their age, were becoming fragile; friends had begun to die. I was entering my fifties, that ambiguous decade marking what's commonly considered in this country the beginning of the end for women. And though I had no less energy or vitality than before, every day it became clearer to me that the world which had grown young behind my back had a different view.

Professor Michael Rutter, a giant among his contemporaries in the field of human development, and his wife Marjorie Rutter, a Nurse Specialist in London, challenge the idea of the crisis as being a developmental *putsch* which occurs at a very specific time in the life span, although they agree that people certainly do have critical times and crises which occur around mid-life. But they explain that while, 'no one doubts that adult life brings with it a host of stresses, rewards, challenges and transitions, there is a sharp contrast between those theorists who portray life-span development as a progression through inevitable universal transitions and stages, and those who view the sequence as open to major individual variations.'

In other words they are arguing that what we experience at mid-life has more to do with what is going on in our separate, unique lives than with some grand universal design for human development. Whereas other developmentalists with their belief in mid-life as a launch-pad for older age which must be forced to make the leap, are more inclined to the idea of a crisis waiting in the wings for a trigger to launch it.

While there seems to be very wide agreement on mid-life being pitched between forty and sixty, the highly respected psychoanalyst Eliott Jacques talks of the rumblings of something which would have 'the character of crisis' beginning as early as the mid-thirties. He elaborates on this by describing a scenario which, we can easily see, might harbinger a crisis: 'The loss of youth, the faltering of physical powers we have always taken for granted, the fading purpose of stereotyped roles by which we have thus far identified ourselves, the spiritual dilemma of having no absolute answers – any or all of these shocks can give this passage the character of a crisis.'

Many of us will have gone through crisis times already in life, perhaps in reaction to some failed ambition or desire, the loss of someone or something very close, but these will have happened within the pattern of that part of life which embodies the goals and tasks of early adulthood and which is still about striving to create a life, even if at times it cannot be adequately done, according to a pattern laid down for us as we move on from childhood and adolescence. The mid-life critical times and actual crisis happen outside that framework. As we enter the middle years there are no such clearly defined goals or aspirations. What we are faced with is drawing up a plan for the future, or at least trying to make some sense of the shapeless, formless oasis it may seem to be, at a time when many of us had assumed a new agenda would be there for us. Discovering a void instead, knowing that we must fill that void with what we have been and hope to become can seem immensely daunting.

Psychologist Sharafat Siddiqui has studied the tensions and reactions to mid-life in his native India and compared it with the experience in the West. He says: 'In my culture where we have very clear stages for each age and the eldest are the most esteemed and in many ways envied, there is a view of some desirable place we aspire to and we believe that older people are the ones able to find that place. This quite obviously makes a great difference to feelings in the middle years. As a boy I can remember well longing to have grey hair and a face full of wise wrinkles. And in India when you reach the time when duties as a parent have ended, then there is a time of assessment to see the purpose of the life we are leading, how it may be used to help others, and how the spiritual dimension can be developed. When this is done it gives people a way to travel and they can prepare for their end and the next life. They may suffer some tensions and problems but they are not the profound crises of identity I see in the West where a measure of success in older age is too often how many material goods have been amassed, how large your name is written on the door at work. These things do not give any guidance as to how to become an elder with a new dimension on life. It doesn't help people find their spirituality. Instead they simply face the knowledge that age is leading to an end. No wonder people cannot cope well with that.'

By contrast, says Dr Fry, we in the West face:

The terrifying awareness of biological time chundering on – it is the unstoppable cycle of living organisms and it sets off some kind of biographical play-through in which we are living out our own drama. There is a mismatch between this natural process which might, in some circumstances bring a sense of moving on and there being important tasks ahead, with what our culture is saying to us. We are surrounded by denial of our mortality. The greatest compliment you can pay someone is to say you do look young instead of, say, you look fifty and nice with it, isn't it good that you are where you are in life. And along with the denying is merit for those who defy the process. You hear people of fifty-five being praised for still getting into the office at seven am instead of praise for the person wise enough to have cut back their hours so that they are learning to be a more thoughtful, tranquil person.

The thing that happens in the experience of Dr Fry is that: 'People outline a blueprint for their lives in the early teens or twenties with goals to be achieved and they drive themselves from then on. Those goals are ever more discordant with the reality of the flesh.'

So when we reach mid-life having lived this way and find we are not high-tech people who can go on and on we become ill with physical symptoms which underlie profound depression. 'When this happens', Dr Fry believes, 'we must grapple with the looming question of how to live the next bit of life in a way that will not go on damaging us.'

These views from the consulting rooms of those asked for help by people struggling with the pains and dilemmas of mid-life are illuminating, and we may be helped to understand why what can feel an entirely random aberration of the spirit, is in fact one of the ways in which we deal with the transition we must make at this stage in life. An impressive number of developmentalists and psychological theorists have set out to show the mid-life time as a step – and a vital one – in our on-going human development. Shakespeare was prescient in talking of the seven stages of man, for the concept of us as progressing from infancy to old age through a series of life stages has been very widely adopted in the past two centuries.

Pre-eminent among those who have divided life into such a pattern was Erik Erikson, a leading figure in the field of psychoanalysis and human development. In his clinical practice he studied the process of growing up in a variety of cultural and social settings. He began with children then moved on to consider how we, as adults, also have a continuing process of development. He constructed a theory of eight stages dividing life from babyhood to old age. His theory will be familiar to our generations, living in the time of high-tech computer games where tasks must be completed in order that we can move on to the next stage. Erikson believed that at different times in life there are particular tasks we must tackle and deal with in order to achieve 'ego integrity' – a state of harmony with ourselves. The value of his work was acknowledged when Erikson was christened 'the father of adult development' by followers and admirers after he published his theory on these eight stages. He was among the first to discuss the transition from middle age to older age as an actual part of our psychological progress. At mid-life we reach the 'adult-hood' phase, he explained, when our task is to assimilate life's experiences, come to accept ourselves, what we have done and where we are in life. Those of us who have come to the middle years have reached a turning point and we are faced with a new set of choices and the tasks we face are in negotiating these choices.

But, as with the computer game which is designed to throw obstacles in our way and test our mettle, so making this transition in real life can be challenging indeed. As Erikson saw it the task we face at this middle point is to turn away from living by an ego which has usefully propelled us so that we made our way in the world as young adults, when we needed the cut and thrust that being driven by the ego gives us to carve our way. But at mid-life, Erikson believed, we must in effect put our immediate egocentric needs on the back burner and begin preparing to take on the immensely important role of an elder in society, qualified to pass on knowledge and wisdom to the next generation.

When we look at it like this it makes sense and seems so clearly right, and yet it is not so simple. We live in a society so focused on youth that it is hard to see what role an elder has these days. It is rare to find older people being asked for their knowledge. How often, for example, do serious television pro-grammes with a question and answer agenda include elders? When do we see them being invited to tell us about the things they know and we do not? Where is there veneration for what our seniors have experienced and learnt in life? When news-papers and weighty magazines carry articles discussing any-thing from news events to philosophical questions about the state of our society, it is far more likely that some bright young arriviste on the adult scene, with a couple of fashionable degrees, will be asked to pontificate. But we must find a way to grow old with conviction. Erikson talks of how, if we cannot make the transition with integrity – a sense of harmony with ourselves – then we may indeed experience despair.

When he was in his mid-forties, Daniel Levinson was motivated to carry out his research looking at the way men aged between thirty-five and forty-five dealt with their maturing. He had been shocked, as he moved into his forties, to discover that, seemingly quite suddenly and without his fully realizing it, a change had taken place and he was no longer seen to be part of a younger generation which, in his own mind, was where he belonged. He expressed how bad it felt when writing his book, *The Seasons of a Man's Life*, which he based on his research: 'Adults hope that life begins at forty – but the great anxiety is that it ends there. In late adulthood a man can no longer occupy the center of his world . . . Moving out of center stage can be traumatic.'

Yet through the work he went on to do, focusing on what may be constructive and positive about ageing, Levinson conceived a ladder-like progression where each step we achieve takes us to a place of higher consciousness as we make our way through 'inevitable universal transitions and stages'. Through this work Levinson came to see middle adulthood as the crucial generation where we have 'dominance' in career and family, explains writer Betty Friedan who was a student alongside Levinson at Berkeley, when he was conducting his research. And looking further ahead than his research had taken him – it ended in the fifties – Levinson echoed Erikson in saying that development at the end of life means coming to terms with the self – knowing it and loving it reasonably well.

I am drawn to the approach of psychologist Abraham Maslow because I recognize the validity of what he says about the stages of life I have already been through, and on that basis it seems likely that he may provide a useful guide to what I can expect in the next part of life. He built his *hierarchy of needs* theory around the idea that we are driven to fulfil whatever the most pressing needs are at different stages in our development. So we seek ways to have hunger and thirst met as our primary need in babyhood and this is followed by the search for security and stability, a sense of belonging. Growing into adulthood we strive to attain love and an identity which allows us a comfortable place in society. When these have been achieved to the best of our abilities we concern ourselves with building self-esteem and self-respect, often through tangible and demonstrable things like career, earning power, gaining status. In other words we try to find a way to have our needs fulfilled through society's mirroring of our worth. It is only then, when these needs have been met and we have been able to assimilate our experiences, accept who we are and achieve a sense of completeness – a similar goal to that set up by Erikson – that we achieve the top of the hierarchy and what Maslow called 'self-actualization'. This he saw as the ultimate goal and he too held that there is a developmental impulse which is stronger than our rational thought, pushing us to work our way up the *hierarchy of needs* even when we may be using all our rational powers to resist.

It has been interesting to watch, among my peers, as we struggle with mid-life issues, how many are beginning to look for a way to find spiritual strength, a quieter kind of satisfaction than perhaps they sought in earlier times. C. G. Jung devoted many years of his adult life to exploring the mind, reaching for a spiritual way of living, and his writings are full of his own quest to achieve this. In searching for a way of making sense of the tumult people so often feel in middle-life, Jung pointed to the similarities between this and second adolescence: 'It is a sort of second puberty, not infrequently accompanied by tempests of passion, the dangerous age.' Just as the pubescent boy or girl has to cast off the dependencies and special pleading of childhood in order to become an independent and effective adult, so we, reduced very often to emotional kids, must find a way to stop looking backwards and measuring ourselves by what has been, and look to who and what we can become.

So we who have already lived a substantial chunk of life might do well to review our lives thus far and, almost as we might paste-up a family album, bring together our memories and experiences and package them so that they can be drawn on and validated in times ahead.

I suspected when I embarked on this book that women would be more prone to mid-life critical times than men because women have certain obviously painful occurrences to act as triggers. The empty-nest syndrome may be more acute for a mother than for a father, if she has spent a lot more time with her children than he has and this, of course, is still by far the commonest pattern. More women than men appear to be left by a partner in the middle years, and often for a younger woman. Women must go through the menopause with all the feelings that may bring about being less of a sexual person as well as it being a very clear signal of ageing, and women more often than men must sacrifice independence or a career to act as carer to a sick person.

But as I set out to interview men, I realized how wrong I was – I had failed to understand how profoundly men fear the loss of their youth, the fear of being without the identity work provides and of no longer keeping up with younger men both at work and as a sexual being. A considerable number find their sexual prowess failing and men too may be left by a partner, although it is less likely to be for a younger man. Men suffer as their children leave home, although, as will be discussed later, it may be for different reasons from women. These can all be powerful triggers to male critical times. Although men are more inclined to keep quiet in public about what is happening, it seems that they not only suffer at least as much but are often more fazed and less practised at knowing how to recognize and set about exploring their feelings than women are.

I have talked of the difficulties of acknowledging that we no longer belong in the youth camp as we reach mid-life, but it is also a stage when people find themselves ruminating about their time as a child, and many of us find there is an intense nostalgia for the sense of being cared for and looked after, and of course this is a time when we turn to those older than us, grateful for the expertise and guidance. Childhood is the foundation stone of our lives and at best it is a time when we can be carefree, full of hopes and dreams, a time when life seems infinite. Mid-life, on the other hand, is the era when we have to recognize that childhood is the other side of the bridge from where we are going, and part of what we go through is a mourning process for that time, as well as the fear of the unknown ahead. Few people, in my view, have expressed the realization which comes with the process of growing up and growing older and the recognition that we are alone better than T. S. Eliot in 'East Coker' (*Four Quartets*):

> Home is where one starts from. As we grow older
> The world becomes stranger, the pattern more complicated
> Of dead and living. Not the intense moment
> Isolated, with no before and after.

Lisa, coming up for fifty, regularly has vivid images in her mind of herself when young. She says: 'I find myself thinking a lot about how I felt as a small child, and I sometimes feel an almost unbearable longing to just be looked after, to be dependent, to let go of responsibility for everything. But of course I know that if I am dependent again it will be because I've become infirm and can't cope. That's very different to being cared for by someone who has chosen to have you that way.'

Jack, fifty-three, feels: 'It is a struggle letting go of the picture I carry in my mind of myself as someone young and who is entitled to the indulgence children get. I keep expecting people to say "haven't you done well" in the way they do to young people when *they* do something well. Then when I force myself to face reality I feel cheated in some way.'

We hear poignancy in the words of Françoise Sagan, the French writer, contemplating her life at forty-two: 'I wish I were ten again. I wish I weren't an adult.'

Mourning childhood and youth and acknowledging that they are gone is hard enough, but while doing this we must also grapple with the fact that death is a reality which, no matter what skills we have, we cannot duck. And it is this which psychoanalyst Eliott Jacques believes lies at the heart of the mid-life crisis: 'The paradox is that of entering the prime of life, the stage of fulfilment, but at the same time the prime and fulfilment are dated. It is this entry upon the psychological scene of the reality and inevitability of one's own eventual personal death, that is the central and crucial feature of the mid-life phase – the feature which precipitates the critical nature of the period.' Death is something which happens around us to people we know, to peers, to people not that much older. We are brought face to face with mortality at the conscious level, explains Jacques: 'Instead of being a general conception, or an event experienced in terms of the loss of someone else, it becomes a personal matter, one's own death, one's own real and actual mortality.'

We may not necessarily dwell on the idea of mortality, but what does happen is that we become aware, as Levinson did, of a world which has us ear-marked as having moved into the domain of those seen to be moving towards older age. It was attending a conference in New York where people were divided into elders and non-elders which hit psychologist Lane Burleigh, who recognizes the irony of his position offering help to people grappling with their critical times in the middle years, while doing the same himself. He says, 'I had just turned fifty and I had become an elder. I had to come to grips with what the hell that meant. I don't feel like an elder and there seemed little to welcome me into the community of elders. As well as working with older people, I work with kids and I see even at that stage that there are no proper processes leading them through life. Years ago in other cultures you had rituals and initiations that welcomed you from one point of life into another; you would have a forty-day excursion into the desert to fast, and ritual scarring, which led to acceptance by elders. There would be training to turn you into a mature person and then you would finally move into a place in your society which you had earned. Here you turn sixteen, you get a driver's licence. Suddenly you have four thousand pounds of steel you can move around. In America you get drafted into a war or at twenty-one you get to vote and you don't even know what the electoral process is all about. There's no stage by stage development, earning your place in society and being revered for having done so. Quite the opposite, and when I see myself as an elder I see myself on a downhill slope leading to a steady diminution of who I am and then death. It's scary.'

That fear may make us look for ways to feel young again, to convince ourselves we really have not aged even though our contemporaries may very clearly have done so. Psychoanalyst Eliott Jacques did not have any illusions about the resistance we may put up to allowing, if necessary, some kind of breaking down, disintegration of our denial and defensive structures, in order to enable the frightened part of ourselves to accept what must be and work with it. He acknowledges: 'What is simple from the point of view of chronology is not simple psychologically. The individual has stopped growing up and has begun to grow old.'

We may recognize in ourselves or others the horrified reaction to this situation in John Updike's 'Rabbit' character Harry Angstrom, whose licentious and self-gratifying existence was the motivation for keeping going in life. When age saps his energy, and even his lust, and eventually lands him with a heart attack so that in *Rabbit Run* Angstrom is in his mid-fifties in a state of flailing helplessness, a man who cannot bear his own ageing, caught, pathetic, like a fly on sticky paper unable to see a way to get beyond the yearning to be the man he was two decades ago.

That is rather the way it was for Mark Gerzon who observes,

looking back, how thoroughly his lifestyle as a 'personality' in California, had him living in a way which meant denying his ageing or bust. It took a profound crisis of the soul, he says, to get him examining where he was in life and how much harm his addiction to being the young blade was doing him. It was a case, he reflects, of addressing the despair he felt. In doing so he re-framed what he believes was a classic mid-life crisis as 'a mid-life quest'. He says: 'At the beginning of the second half of life I had started to feel old, I had started to feel tired. I had started to feel the imminence of death, I had started to feel that nothing made any difference, including any of my successes. One might say that's depression but it wasn't. It was the beginning of my re-examination of the rules of the first half of life.'

This process takes people in different directions and at its most extreme may be as drastic as radically changing everything in their life. A process of stripping away the appendages, the status, the possessions of the first part of life may seem imperative. That process leading us to some kind of renewal is brought to us vividly in the actions of Friedrich Klein the protaganist of Hermann Hesse's novella *Klein and Wagner*:

Yes, he had once been young, and no commonplace youth; he had dreamed great dreams, had asked much of life and of himself. But since then there had been nothing but dust and burdens, the long road, heat and weary legs, and a slumberous, ageing nostalgia lurking in his parching heart. That had been his life. That had been his life.

Now Klein could read a part of the signpost of his destiny. He was leaving behind his marriage, his job, everything which had hitherto been life and homeland to him . . . And in doing this he had fulfilled the most glowing dream of his youth, that youth whose relics had vanished along the dreary road of a meaningless life.

Most people do not choose so drastic a way, but some do. This is how it was for George Goldschmidt, fifty-two, a Dutchman who also left a life with all the things we judge as a source of satisfaction: a wife and children, an interesting and

successful career in business, money to buy comfort and opportunities for travel. Friends envied him. He smiles, a twist of the
lips, wryly mocking himself: 'I was a very successful businessman – it seemed I had the Midas touch and everything I
embarked on went well. I got a tremendous kick out of this. I
was living fast, and very much for show. I assumed that the
harder I worked, the bigger the business grew the better my
life would be. I had eleven offices around the world. I was
married with two young children whom I adored and we had
what everyone thought a rather good life.'

Except that it did not feel like such a good life to George: 'I
was like a great echoing, hollow drum, great to beat a tune on
but there was nothing inside to give depth to that tune. I had
such a sense of futility and there seemed no way of changing
that. The only thing I could think of was to change everything
in the hope it would fill the hollow and make me feel different.
I divorced my wife and nobody could understand why because
we had seemed fine. I quit the business without any plan other
than to try to find a way of living that made more sense.'

For a while George travelled a bit, drank a good deal, got
involved with business deals again and began to experience
feelings of panic because still nothing made sense. It was
during this time that he met someone who had lived at the
spiritual community Findhorn in the north of Scotland. He
says: 'I took myself off to live there. I began working as a
kitchen hand, living in a wooden hut and feeling terrified for
quite a time at the lack of pressure and deadlines, at having so
few demands on me. But that changed.'

A similar sense of emptiness and futility on reaching mid-
life, and the feeling that there must be a way to discover more
within himself led David Lyons, in his mid-fifties, to become
'an unfaithful, constantly questioning man so unlike the person
I had known before'. He had married in his twenties and he
and his wife had a daughter who delighted them. They now
also have grandchildren close by. He says: 'My wife and I had
a great sense of purpose for the first twenty years. We worked

together, shared values it seems, and although my wife never liked sex much, somehow there was so much to be done, so many goals to meet that it only sometimes upset me. But as our daughter left home the perspective seemed to shift. My wife appeared to become more interested in proving she could do better at the work we shared in catering than I could, and far less interested in our relationship. I began to feel an absolute yearning for warmth, passion to let that bit of me which seemed totally squashed come alive again. I began to think about leaving but then my wife became ill and that seemed to make the whole idea impossible.'

Instead he went on a two-week fiction writing course where he tells: 'I seemed to be unleashed. I started writing and writing, getting feedback from the group and my ego soared. I appeared to be popular, I had a sudden sense that life could be like this, and of course it was then that I fell madly and wildly in love with a woman, not a younger woman, she was close to my own age, and the thing I couldn't believe was that I, the middle-aged sensible chap I was viewed as in my home town, was caught up in this extraordinary reality. I remember the first time this woman and I made love I was in her room, stroking her back and she turned over, put her finger on my lips and said: "Don't talk, just make love to me." I seemed to have a power, a potency, the ability to delight her. The contrast with how I felt then as though the future were a magical possibility made going back to my ordinary life very difficult.

'But there's not an easy answer – certainly just leaving isn't it. For the time being I am putting a lot of emotion into my writing, as a way of pushing away the immediacy of the pain, and I've managed to change things so that I have more time for myself, more independence and although it's not ideal I don't feel I want to leave my wife and nor do I want to be one of those men who has a lot of affairs on the side. I see now that I have to try to find a way of experiencing that passion and delight in life which I glimpsed in some other way. But I'm not quite there yet.'

Relationships are likely to feel, as much as anything, the impact of critical times. It is the central relationship, the thing which once seemed the central support to life, within which it was possible to fulfil dreams and develop, which can come to seem a prison at mid-life. Dissatisfaction with work, disillusion with what has been achieved, a sense that life does not add up to the expectations, a sense of failure, can very easily be blamed on a partner and on the quality of what goes on within the relationship. Familiarity, comfort, a well-worn pattern of communication can come to seem deadening and uninteresting, the reason we are not as vibrant, full of libido, as stimulated or stimulating as we remember ourselves being when younger. And the ticking of the clock in the background to our lives brings a sense of panic and urgency: will we ever feel super-stimulated, high with excitement again; if we do not move fast will it not be too late for any opportunities to occur? The fear that transcendental feelings will never be experienced again can seem unbearable.

As we have seen with George and David, men are inclined to see the relationship which they feel should answer all their emotional questions, as the problem, the source of what is wrong with them, when they have the kind of desperate empty feelings described here. It is not at all uncommon for them to convince themselves that they should leave in the belief that they will experience something more authentic on their own or in another relationship.

It was precisely this belief which led Michael to walk out on his wife of twenty years and his two teenage children so that he could live with a woman he had met through work. He sits opposite me in a chair telling his story and I watch the confident, assertive man who came in become quieter and sadder as he talks until, by the end of our conversation, there are tears running down his cheeks.

Michael explained but did not attempt to justify having behaved in a way which clearly devastated his children, as well as his wife, a great deal. He says: 'I was in a vulnerable state at the time. I had been made unemployed from a prestigious job and it was a shock to find that getting the same kind of work to replace it wasn't easy. It threw me into turmoil. Suddenly the things which had seemed secure and right in my life before, seemed a burden. I really was aware of feeling trapped, bored and frightened, and my wife wasn't able to do anything to help me. It wasn't her fault of course, but all the same I felt the ordinariness of our lives was sapping my energy and ability to be dynamic enough to get work.'

He might, he thinks, have coped with that if, at the same time, he had not recognized very clearly that he was ageing. 'I saw myself getting old, I had a very graphic picture in my mind of myself as an old bent man on a road leading in an unchanging way into nothingness. I felt horror, panic, utter misery at this and nothing in my life seemed to sustain or make sense.'

As so often happens Michael turned to another woman, in his case at work, who offered an understanding of his state: 'All the unhappiness from the past and my fear of the future, which I hadn't realized was so close to the surface came up. This woman recognized in me the little boy who had not been hugged by his mother, who never felt loved, and at that time when I was feeling so wretched I so much wanted some loving and understanding. Gina seemed to offer that. It was her insights, the things she said to me, which seemed terribly significant and I simply felt I would die if I couldn't be with her.' But as he said all this Michael began almost compulsively to describe the scene when he told his wife he was going. 'She was standing brushing her hair and I told her I felt I had to go and that our marriage was not going to allow either of us to develop. She just hit me with the brush over and over again and then our sixteen-year-old daughter heard the noise and came in. Then my fourteen-year-old boy Robbie came in and I told him too. It was terrible how upset they all were.'

Telling the tale he can see the brutality of it all but he talks of what he did as a compulsion: 'I had no idea what I was doing, what I was inflicting on my children when I left and the guilt I have been through is enormous. Of course it's had its effect on my relationship with Gina. I killed the joy in what we had. I hadn't realized that you can't cause such a lot of pain and then go on and live happily in a carefree way. I don't know what will happen with Gina and me but it's shaky right now and the irony is when I look back I think my marriage to Louise wasn't bad at all and perhaps I could have found a different way to try to grow. But it's too late . . .'

Fifty-year-old Richard Levenson's trajectory was very similar, but he feels he was right to find the courage to change things at that mid-life stage. He had lived 'the life which was expected of me, a good Jewish boy. I married. I went into business – advertising – repressing the thing I really wanted which was to be a sculptor. My wife had tolerated my attempts at sculpture but she had never been more than mildly amused by it and I did not feel I could progress with it while we were together. Our marriage had been held together by our mutual involvement with our sons, but they had left, and I was trapped with feeling empty and bleak but also suffocating. Some days I really felt I would die if I did not get away and express the person I wanted to be. So my wife and I separated which was traumatic – the exploding of a family with all the pain that involves for everyone.

'But I think at fifty you have a sense that you had better do something, that there's an awful lot to get on with. I do believe when you hit sixty you have to start accepting your life and realizing that it is reaching towards the end and that nobody but you can work things out for that final bit.

I did wonder at the time if I had any right to be so destructive. But I am now sure it was the right thing to do because my kids are beginning to see something new, much more alive in me, even though they are still angry as hell. I have confidence that we will all have a better future than if I had stayed.'

There are other reasons, of course, why relationships teeter and collapse at this stage. When a partnership has been shaped too thoroughly around children it may seem devoid of life and stimulus after they have gone and partners find they have no idea how to relate as just a couple any longer. I will explore the empty-nest syndrome as it is called, further on. Another cause of difficulties can be a shifting power balance in a relationship. For example a wife who has been very absorbed in her domestic role, who, perhaps, has been content to take a subservient role, may at this time start wanting to do things for herself. Many women in mid-life re-train for work or begin studying, others develop hobbies which take them into new circles of friends. When such things happen a man who is, possibly, finding it hard to keep up at work or who feels sexually less potent than in earlier days, can feel that he is losing his place in the family and become upset or angry.

The statistics on marriages ending in later life (living-together arrangements are not recorded) make distressing reading. The destruction of lives interwoven together with years of intimacy is something which Renate Olins, Director of the London Marriage Guidance Council sees over and over again. Between the ages of forty and fifty-nine approximately 32 per cent of couples separate – that is one-third of partnerships, most of which have probably endured the stresses and trials of rearing a family and establishing a way of being together. Olins says: 'It is a moment when people review their lives. Having stayed together in a marriage which was not necessarily all that happy, they cast around for other options. And the present generations reaching mid-life have grown up believing powerfully in individual fulfilment. That is a nice catch-phrase but the price of it can be very high.'

It is not surprising that it is infidelity which often splits the fragile mid-life marriage. A partner feeling frightened, trapped, that there is no possibility of the excitement they crave within the long-term relationship, will very often see another relationship as the solution. And of course it is true that, in the short term at least, there is little like the heady passion and intensity of feeling that an affair with a new lover can bring. It can indeed seem the solution and for mid-lifers there may be a feeling of greater urgency, of the need to seize the hour, than younger people experience.

Almost as many women as men now commit adultery, according to Annette Lawson whose large research study *Adultery* showed a steady upward trend among both sexes, and other research has suggested more recently that the pattern is the same. There does, however, appear to be a difference in what men and women look for in an affair. American author Dalma Heyn in her book *The Erotic Silence of the Married Woman* found that many women incorporated a secret long-term lover into their married life as a way of tolerating and staying with their husbands.

Bonnie Norton, a publicist in her early fifties, talked of how, in the past, she had 'turned away from opportunities for infidelity' but when she met a man who offered passion but also took pleasure in her company during the mid-life years when she felt at a low ebb, she explained: 'I felt drawn, almost as though I had no control over what was happening.' And she justified it expressing a sentiment repeated frequently: 'My partner treated me like a household fixture – at least that is how it seemed to me. This really felt like a last chance. I couldn't imagine being able to attract lovers as I got older.'

She remembers the way she rationalized her affair: 'My partner had been very involved in himself, his own interests and way of life and although he was good with our two daughters, I felt utterly worthless. I think I was extremely angry about this although I never voiced it. That anger had turned into a kind of depressed acceptance.

'It was by chance that I met Sam at a seminar I attended and he listened to what I had to say, seemed fascinated and clearly fancied me. It was heady stuff for a forty-six-year-old woman feeling like a has-been. We met a few times and the chemistry between us was enormous – we were like a couple of magnets forever being drawn together. I couldn't believe I was allowed this wonderful treat. The really compelling thing was it made me feel so special and so young. I felt invulnerable.'

Affairs can seem a solution because the married person going into one has not considered what the outcome will have to be. But usually after a time people either feel they must do something about the relationship or it must end, so that there will be the enormous upheaval either of breaking off with the spouse, or of coping with the pain. It is not surprising that a person suffering in this way either shows too clearly what is wrong so that the affair is discovered this way or focuses the cause of the pain on the husband or wife whom they see as having pushed them into the affair, thus causing all the pain.

If an affair is confessed or discovered it will have repercussions which few people anticipate as they embark on the liaison. Psychologist Janet Reibstein, co-author with psychologist Martin Richards of *Sexual Arrangements*, a study of how people manage infidelity, has seen how discovering that a partner has had an affair may well lead to him or her having their own crisis. In any event, she explains, relationships are never the same after an affair has been revealed. She describes how 'the pattern is either that the couple's long-term relationship falls apart. This may not happen immediately, but later as the shattering impact of what has happened sinks in. Or, if the relationship does survive and both partners have committed themselves to keeping it together, you can be certain, there will be a new dynamic and that is something they need to be aware of and to deal with.'

This was the experience of Georgina Wall who discovered that for many of the thirty years she had been married to her husband, he had had a mistress he did not want to give up and who had threatened suicide. Georgina moved out of the home and began divorce proceedings. She recalls, 'I had failed to read the signs so the information arose out of the blue. It was a time of anguish, of turmoil, of pre-emptive strikes and rapid decisions, and two of our adult children were having deeply distressing problems of their own just then.'

Her husband then lost his job, career and status because of the affair which was with a work colleague and became depressed. At this point, says Georgina, 'He moved in with me, in my new home, after a brief separation which both of us found unbearable. Since that ghastly period we have been picking up the pieces although there is still blood on the floor and the task has been harder than I could possibly have imagined.'

The new strength Georgina gained through what she regards as a very real crisis allowed her to feel far more separate from her husband, to set limits as to what she would accept in future, in a way she had not been able to do before. In her case the behaviour of her husband precipitated what happened, but that, as she acknowledges, was a symptom of the state their marriage had reached.

If, as women, we grow up believing there is absolute virtue in putting our own needs and achievements behind those of others and if self-denial becomes the way we learn to function – and may even choose to function – after marriage and becoming mothers, it can be very difficult in later life to draw on spirit or conviction about ourselves in order to start visualizing a constructive future.

This is something which Jungian analyst Clarissa Pinkola Estes believes is a key reason why women at mid-life so often come to her wondering what is wrong, why they feel so helpless and hopeless. She talks of how thoroughly these women deny their own needs and desires through the earlier years and 'give dominion over their passionate, creative instinctive life' in order to have marriage, children, a home.

Estes has written a lengthy book, *Women Who Run With the Wolves*, taking mythical stories as the basis of a therapy with women which involves telling stories, drawing on myths and symbol to help them understand their predicament, and as a way of moving forward feeling good about themselves. The style of Estes' writing is in itself mystical and ornate and would not offer guidance to those who choose a more temporal

way of addressing issues. This said, I find considerable sense in
what she is saying, at heart, about the way women give up
supremacy in their lives then reach a point when that position
is becoming less and less likely tυ be a valid one or one which
fits the second stage of life in which there will be far less
context for her subjugation. Estes uses the predicament of a
client to illustrate how she, in the role of therapist, led this
woman to understand what had happened to her.

I worked with a woman who was quite taken advantage of by
others, be they spouse, children, mother, father or stranger. She was
forty years old, and still at this bargain/betrayal stage of inner
development. The poor bargain she had made was to never say no in
order to be consistently loved. The predator of her own psyche
offered her the gold of being loved if she would give up her instincts
that said 'enough is enough'. She realized fully what she was doing
to herself when she had a dream that she was on her hands and
knees in a crowd, trying to reach through the forest of legs for a
precious crown someone had thrown into a corner.
    The instinctual layer of her psyche was pointing out to her that
she had lost her sovereignty over her own life, and that it was going
to be hands-and-knees work to get it back. To get her crown back,
this woman had to re-evaluate her time, her giving her attentions to
others.

Wendy Rhodes might not have expressed it this way, but
she is very clear that she had sacrificed a vital sense of her own
potential and spirit in order to care for the two daughters she
had with the man she married when in her twenties. She
waited until she was sixty and her daughters were settled in
the outside world before she felt able to leave a husband who,
she says, made her feel 'shrunken and tyrannized'. She describes
it as one of the hardest things she had ever done when it came
to it, but it was 'a bid for survival'.
    She explained: 'I didn't realize how deeply depressed I was
until I got away. I went on a visit to America to see a friend
and it was a thrilling experience. Then on the journey back I
thought I'd caught a cold, but it didn't get better and I was off

work for a long time. I have now been told by a doctor that it was a manifestation of chronic depression. A lot of things were going on subconsciously. I had never consciously planned to leave my husband, but it was just that at a certain moment I knew I couldn't stay. I was gripped with an absolute desperation, I had to get out. I packed the boot of the car and phoned my husband at work to say I was going. He came looking for me but I managed to stay with friends he didn't know. People thought I was very cruel; my husband was on the point of retirement, they said he was going to seed and drinking too much after I had gone. But at that time I had the clearest picture of two divergent paths and I had to choose one. The one where I was alone looked scary and lonely but there was a sense of hopefulness, if I stayed on the other path I saw myself with my husband but shrivelling up and dying.'

Yet it can also be fear of no longer having anybody to give attentions to, which precipitates one of the most familiar crises, and it is far more often women than men who experience this. The empty-nest syndrome, as it is called, may feel devastating. But a time that can be equally painful although less acknowledged as such, is that period when children are preparing themselves for independence. Throughout later adolescence they let us know how keen they are to be free and to live their own lives and they may do this in a way which makes us feel terribly rejected and turned against. Suddenly, after years of knowing we were needed and depended upon, that we were the centrepiece in their lives, we find ourselves increasingly relegated to what feels like a bit part in the lives our children are planning and building for themselves.

It can be very hurtful and we may, because of our feelings of being rejected and undervalued, hurt ourselves further by becoming angry, bitter even, with children who seem so utterly egocentric, so ungrateful for all we have done. Yet this is a perfectly normal stage, and in truth our role as parent continuing to offer the support, the security our children need in order to be able to be independent, is vital.

But standing back in an entirely adult way and recognizing this may not be easy. Those of us who are already feeling dread and sadness at the prospect of our children departing may find all sorts of panicky fears of loneliness; we may question how sense will be made of life ahead. Psychoanalyst Dinora Pines knows well how deep the sadness of potential loss can go and acknowledges: 'For women who have had children, depression may be linked to the children's adolescence, to their struggle to separate from the parents which eventually leads to their leaving home.'

The way Meg Brown, who at forty-six was preparing for her eldest son to leave for a volunteer job in India, felt, was echoed many times over in the conversations I had with women. She expressed it this way: 'I look at my children and see their eagerness to be out in the world, testing their strength, exploring possibilities, and having adventures. In one way I feel very proud that they are so excited by life, but I also feel terribly discarded. My husband doesn't feel it like this. He is pleased the kids have grown up feeling confident about the world and doesn't seem to feel the sense of rejection I do at what I suppose is their change of focus. I feel them pulling away from me a little more every day. I can't say to them "Look after me, I feel scared and frightened of the loneliness ahead", because that's not on with kids, but I wish they would show that I still matter to them. It's not easy being a parent who is so clearly needed and wanted one minute and to find, the next minute it seems, that you are almost irrelevant except as the person providing a secure base. I sometimes think how much they've got and how little I seem to have ahead by comparison. I know that's probably stupid but it's how it feels.'

One of the things that happens when our children appear this way and when we feel vulnerable and unsure about life is that the child-parent relationship is inverted, so that the parent or parents are looking to their young, even when they try hard not to do so, for succour, while the children, sensing a dependency they do not want, may become even more urgent in their attempts to push their parents away. When this is happening it is very difficult to recognize that children in this state still do need their parents and although the circumstances may change they will, unless the relationship is so damaged that love and caring have actually gone, probably continue to want them and to keep a strong contact. But none of this appears likely or comforting when homes are full of the breaking of childhood bonds and for parents struggling with their own mid-life feelings and issues it is absolutely understandable that the feelings around the emptying nest are acute.

None of this is made easier by the fact that these emotions may very well be experienced alongside the turbulence of dealing with the mercurial emotions, the argumentativeness, the pushing for ever more rights within the domestic sphere which many young display when they are at the betwixt and between stage of reaching for autonomy but at the same time going through their own fears and uncertainties at what lies ahead. Apparent confidence and eagerness to be out and free is frequently acted out at home in fluctuating moods, sweet closeness one minute, the behaviour of an arch-enemy the next.

The difficulty for those of us going through this stage is that, while we will probably be offered condolence and may feel able to seek help if we are very unhappy when children have actually gone and we are experiencing the empty nest, our distress can seem far less acceptable when children are preparing to leave yet are still at home. People tend to try to point to the advantages of children having gone, but no amount of listening to others as we try to imagine how we will fill the gaps, what it will mean when our children's rooms remain tidy, the decibel count is tolerable, friends do not hammer on the door for half the night, will necessarily dull the fear. There is lots of gung ho stuff around telling us to take up flamenco dancing and befriend needy kids but it misses the point so utterly that if anything the intended kindness is alienating.

What we have to face is the difficult truth that our kids have moved on, we will no longer be centre stage in their lives, we cannot reclaim that era when being a parent was our primary role. It may seem at this time that our children are going forth, maybe slightly hesitantly, but nevertheless towards a future which leads uphill while ours may seem at this time to lead at best towards an empty plateau and at worst downhill. This is certainly not the way it need be and many parents bear testimony to the fact that the moment can in fact be as liberating as it is full of loss, but we do not necessarily find that out immediately. First we may indeed have to go through a process of mourning the departure of the young around whom we have shaped so many years of our lives, in order to discover the pleasures of having time for ourselves.

Dorothy Little has just turned fifty, she has an administrative job at a school, which she thoroughly enjoys, and she thought she had prepared herself well to withstand her daughter's departure for university: 'I had my career, I do a bit of volunteer work which I enjoy, and I have a good social life. I'd always been aware I needed to have some separate life from my children's and I felt I had done that. In fact I remember Becky saying to me at times that I was selfish because I was always wrapped up in my own life. So nothing prepared me for my desperate grief in the days after she had gone away because she was the last. Somehow when the other two went I just focused on Becky so I didn't feel the emptiness the same way, but this time was tough. The worst thing was going to Sainsbury's and realizing I didn't need to do a proper shop because there was only me to feed, and I found six in the evening awful because that was the time I used to start making supper, and suddenly there was no need.

'It's nine months now since she went and I have found the adjustment difficult, but I have worked hard at doing it. I started making dates with friends for several evenings a week so that I really didn't have a chance to mope and it was fun. I had forgotten how enjoyable and what good support it is being with friends. I have men and women friends and I've come to value them so much the past months. I also signed up for some group weekends away in the country and that was interesting – one was a disaster because I didn't get on at all with the other people, but that didn't matter, it was an experience. I still miss Becky around the place but not in the way I did before where I kept thinking of her and finding tears in my eyes. Now I look forward to seeing her in the holidays but I can see that my life is very pleasant in its new shape.'

But how hard we make it for ourselves by feeling we should be strong and that we should shut up and put up with the pain of all this, that there is something reprehensible in such powerful feelings around the burgeoning independence of our young. We need to be kinder to ourselves, to open up what is, after all, an upsetting experience for so very many people and recognize that by acknowledging and grieving for what has gone, by facing the chilling fear that perhaps the yawning gap in life will never be able to be filled, we can help ourselves to move forward.

Claudia Lewis, now fifty-one, went through an eighteen-month period of mourning which she refused to acknowledge: 'I didn't know why I felt so lost and miserable. I had thought I was ready for the kids to go. My partner and I needed time as just a couple, it seemed absolutely the right thing. It wasn't until somebody pointed out to me that however nice the idea of free time and more space in the house might be, I was having to acknowledge that I had reached an end of time as a mother and that could never come back. Also it had been a very intense period. My husband and I divorced when I was young so I brought the children up on my own; I had quite a hard time looking after their interests and my partner's and then their father died. So we went through a lot together – and that included their adolescence which was a pretty fraught time, but it brought us close. Then suddenly there they were preparing to fly and I was going around saying, "Isn't it great they are growing up?" and wondering why I wanted to burst into tears.'

Rose Robinson, who came to Britain from St Lucia during the 1960s, having lived among her own family until well into adult life, as did her siblings, found it very hard when the last of her five children left home: 'This is like a turning point. It felt terrible. You have to come to terms with it and to say I'll get on with my life. I used to read about it . . . women getting depressed because all the children had flown the nest, and I'd think but you have all the time in the world . . . but then you realize it's a serious thing. I didn't think I'd miss Gemma as much as I do. I go into her room and look at her things. You don't know what it's going to be like, nobody can tell you.'

Because mid-life is a time when we may lose parents, the chance of us experiencing actual bereavement and the end of our role as a parent to dependent children, simultaneously, is real enough and it is hardly surprising that it can precipitate a crisis which spills over into depression or an overwhelming sense of not having done enough with what can feel like the significant part of our lives. In these circumstances the sadness at a child going then seems to become part of the mourning for the dead person. Daphne Berkovi's son left home for university soon after the death of her mother and the intensity of pain certainly felt like another bereavement: 'I was not prepared for such a sad and deep sense of privation; not only had I lost my mother, but I was now losing my son, and my role of mother and home-maker was becoming defunct.' Yet it is also plain that her sadness may have as much to do with a belief that she has wasted opportunities in an irrevocable way as with the moving on of her children: 'Reflections are painful because this brings with it acute feelings of anger and disappointment over wasted years; years when I should have been trying to establish a more diverse lifestyle for myself.'

Similarly Gloria Andrews found the departure of one daughter to college and the marriage of the other not long after the death of a beloved father-in-law devastating: 'I felt very depressed and lonely and my husband couldn't comfort me as he was having his own crisis and retreated into the solace of his computer. I realized I had to try to get on with my own life but whenever I went out shopping I would see mothers with young children and envy them because now I felt entirely alone.'

But what about the men who have fathered these children, if they have been around throughout their growing lives? Is there any reason why they should feel less intensely? If women find it hard to admit to empty-nest feelings, how much harder it may be for men. Psychotherapist and author Susie Orbach believes we need to recognize and validate men's feelings of loss at a child's departure, allowing and indeed encouraging them to share the grieving rather than insisting they are the outsiders to this drama, leaving them to look for other ways to act it out. In an article in the *Guardian* Orbach postulated a father she named James who, she said, 'found himself extremely interested in his young secretary a week after his son had left for university. A large gap threatened his equilibrium because his son had provided much friendship, closeness as well as a link with youth.' James ridiculed his wife's tears, Orbach explained, and compensated for his loss by taking his secretary out and basking in her admiration of him as a mentor – 'an important aspect of his relationship with his son'. In this case his wife, Orbach explained, wisely and bravely confronted James and helped him recognize that she too was suffering. She helped him to see that they could share the experience of getting through the pain and 'rediscover one another and to hold and nurture each other through this phase of life'.

As mothers, it is often our proximity to children which causes the pain when they go, but for men it can be the flipside. If fathers have been absent working long hours, not really involved with the nitty-gritty of their kids' lives they may suddenly realize that their children are ready to go and that they have missed their childhoods. Keith Bremner who runs groups for men in which many come to explore feelings about the kind of parenting they have had and the kind of parents they have been, sees so often a convoluted, hidden grieving which men have not acknowledged: 'Men who have been brought up in a traditional way believing it right to put all their time and energy into work so that they see very little of their children, find it far harder to make sense of the sad empty feelings they have at the empty nest. They don't connect the feelings to the loss of their young which is why some appear to behave so outrageously going off, searching out new lovers, new experiences and apparently having no feeling for their partners at this difficult time.

'So long as the children are at home they feel as though they are there, and there may be a belief which is not of course thought through, that the time will come when they will be more together with them. But then when these men realize their kids are adults who are about to go off to make their own lives, that they have to face not only what they are losing but that they do not have the relationship they want with their children, they may then experience an overwhelming pain and despair because it all seems too late. Or these feelings may come up later, even years later, when the children have been gone for some time.

Men can collapse and be in absolute anguish, they can lose their sense of purpose in life when they realize that they have missed out on time and intimacy with their children, that the years are gone and all they have is a sort of polite friendship with their kids, and a job that may well not be rewarding them as it did in earlier years. It is an intensely sad thing for men when they come to this.

Bremner believes that while there is a good deal of talk these days about the importance of men in families and for their children, there is not really recognition of what the loss of those children can mean for them and he explains how in his groups they focus on this. He says: 'We encourage men to talk to each other about their feelings and through that they may be able to find a way to talk to their children, about how much they care and their own sense of failure at not having been better fathers. There is a great deal of guilt in men at what they have not done. They will bring up all sorts of poignant memories of times they feel they have let their children down and not been there for them and, knowing they cannot go back and make that right, they often get very upset indeed.'

When men recognize their distress they feel it can be a catalyst which pushes them into making the effort they wish they had made earlier. Dan, a freelance film technician, now sixty-one, found himself so full of grief after his son left home and went to live in another part of the country, that he rented a cottage in the same area and went down every weekend. He says: 'I explained to my wife that I wanted to go on my own because I wanted to try to be there as a father to Jim. Because his Mum's always been the one around, the one he's turned to, I felt I'd just be a background figure if she were with me. She understood – she was the one who helped me see why I was so wretched after Jim went – and so I took myself off each Friday evening. Jim certainly didn't want to be with me all the time. He was making a new life and new friends, but I think he was pleased at what I did and we always managed at least a beer and a meal over the weekends and that was a chance to chat. It wasn't deep emotional stuff although we did sometimes talk about his childhood and I let him know how sorry I was I hadn't been there more. I stopped going when he moved to another job in another town, but by that time we had formed a close bond and I feel all right about him being gone now. I think he feels as I do now that we're there for each other.'

Julian Marsden married young because, he now believes: 'I very much needed respite from a difficult childhood. I was seeking warmth, protection and succour, but I was also very wrapped up in building my career as a doctor. My wife and I had four sons but really I didn't have a great deal to do with them. I was around evenings and weekends a certain amount but I wasn't much good at playing football, that sort of thing, and I think it is the hands-on stuff which helps build the intimacy. I left my wife while our sons were still growing up and so I missed their entry into young adulthood and, as so often happens when men leave partners, I really saw very little of the boys and when I did it was quite often strained and difficult.'

It was not until he had been through psychoanalysis and worked on the fury he felt for his authoritarian father who, Julian believes, 'manipulated me into taking up medicine and taught me to repress feelings and desires', that he began to realize how thoroughly he had lost his children. 'I had gone on a quest for my own fulfilment and at the time that seemed an important enough reason to go. Later, I felt aware of a sense of loss but I did all I could to push it down. But when I went into therapy because I was very unhappy and could not put my finger on why, what it was all about, I started to feel those things that had been repressed. I began to feel great sadness at having missed my children's lives and at what they must have felt. I began trying to build a relationship with them. It was not easy because, of course, they were angry with me and it's taken several years. Now they are grown up we are establishing a friendship as adults and that is rewarding.'

It is quite natural that a big change such as children leaving home, which means a re-organization and re-definition of our lives, may entail a painful re-adjustment, but the majority of people, however desperate they may have felt at the time, can look back a few months later and realize that they *have* adjusted even if they still feel nostalgic for the childhood years.

Claudia Lewis who, earlier, talked of her distress at the departure, began to fill the extra time she had with researching a story which had long fascinated her and writing it up. She left a full-time job teaching music and went freelance which enabled her to take on just the projects which really interested her. She says, 'I began to enjoy life in a new way and that was a wonderful antidote to the children going, but in truth it took eighteen months before I felt I really was pleased that they were out in the world and I had life for myself and my partner.

In fact when my daughter came back temporarily I didn't feel all that pleased. It wasn't right for her, I felt, and in truth I didn't want to get sucked back into the maternal role.'

Professor Sir Michael Rutter and Marjorie Rutter also found that the reality of the empty nest need not be traumatic unless we have so built our lives around our children that we are too emotionally dependent upon them, requiring them to fulfil our emotional needs in an inappropriate way. They point to research in which 160 women, on average in their mid-forties, with children in various stages of leaving home, were interviewed and they conclude: 'The great majority viewed the impending or actual departure of their children with a sense of relief, albeit mixed with some ambivalence.'

If we do grieve so deeply that it turns to depression it may be worth seeking help in the view of therapist Diana Glassner, who sees this grief in her consulting room. She says: 'There may be feelings from our own childhood tangled up in what we feel about losing our children; it may be that our children have protected us from the world outside and now we are very scared at the prospect of having to do as we see our children doing and go out into the world and make our way. We may indeed have put all our love and emotion into the children and find ourselves suddenly faced with a relationship that is hollow because of this, and we are terrified.'

There are different kinds of help we can turn to if we want to try to unravel or tackle our grief. Therapy where we explore a past which may provide links and 'explanations' is one way, other therapies help us to express our feelings and look at how we may deal with the immediate pains. Psychological, behavioural, and cognitive methods teach us to modify or change our behaviour in the hope that this will enable us to function in a more constructive way. For others a counsellor who will lead us, in a very practical way, to see how we can restructure our lives may be the help we need. There are people who have been much helped by exercise methods with a spiritual dimension such as yoga and tai chi, or by spiritual therapies. But a depression which does not respond to other methods and will not shift or lift may require the intervention of a doctor.

The critical time for parents when children leave home is one thing, but how do men and women who have not had children and who must, at mid-life, acknowledge that this is something which will not be a part of their life feel? It is a momentous thing to face in a world where the axis of people's lives in any society, is the rearing of children. I think of my good friend who has had two abortions because the pregnancies came at 'impossibly difficult times, in one case with a partner I knew would not be supportive, and at another when I was alone and without money,' but who now, aged forty-eight, feels the pain and loss all the time. She berates herself: 'I so much want a child and I just threw away the possibility. I think of adoption – but I would only get a child with huge difficulties and I'm not sure I can cope with that. I have to find a way to come to terms with living in a positive way without a child.' And, indeed, last time we spoke she had given up a teaching job which sapped all her time and energy and was spending much time painting – a thing which earns her very little money but which she finds a pleasure and solace.

Living without a partner may add to the sense of utter aloneness but even within a relationship, we can also feel quite desperate at seeing the last chance of fertility fade away and it is not surprising that the end of any hope of having children may precipitate a crisis.

When Helen married she had a bright, clear picture in her mind of four children romping in a field surrounded by a white picket fence. Moving to a town in the hills above San Francisco, with its rolling vistas of fields and woodland and further down the pale sandy beach and turquoise sea, was something Helen and her husband Bob did with the children they would have in mind. She remembers every bit of the process of trying to achieve this dream: 'We tried, in the ordinary way, for several years and then I got pregnant at last. We were delighted. I miscarried. I got pregnant again two years later and again there was delight followed by the miscarriage and the same cycle a third time. I began then to think there was something wrong with me but another bit of me felt, in a very bolshie way, that there certainly wasn't anything wrong with me, that I was as good as anyone else and we would keep on trying. So we did and it was awful. Our marriage became very strained and Bob went through all the awful feelings of failure men have in these circumstances. It meant our life was put on hold and our relationship drew further and further apart. I couldn't think about anything else, plan anything for the future, envisage our relationship in the future without children.

'We tried *in vitro* fertilization. The doctors discovered I had a big ovarian cyst so I had to have that taken out. Then there were further operations and I took about thirty drugs in all over a ten-year period. There was a kind of madness in me. I couldn't give up. I think if I had never conceived I might have stopped trying and accepted infertility sooner, but it was the knowledge that it could happen which drove me on. And of course doctors don't discourage you because there is a lot of money in it, so I wasn't faced with looking at how low the chances of success were but rather the chance that I might just end up with a baby.

'Bob was immensely supportive and kind but he didn't talk about it much. I had to have these injections every day with a drug to induce the ovaries to produce eggs and Bob used to give me the injections and when I was going to have an examination I had to drive to the city with his sperm in the car, get to the doctor's office, and then they had to wash it and get all the bacteria out before inseminating it right into the uterus. I did that for several months and it was feverish and mad.

'By the time I reached forty I was utterly exhausted and at the end of my tether and this doctor, a wonderful English doctor in San Francisco, sat me down and said, "Just give yourself a break. You've done everything and there's no sense in trying again." He pointed out that only 20 per cent of people get pregnant with *in vitro*, that it puts your body through so much and costs a fortune. And he just talked to me about thinking positively about a life I could have without children, that perhaps it wasn't the only thing which would make life worthwhile. I remember he said "Let it go. That's what you have to do now." I am still grateful to that man. He got me off a mad jag I was on and which was wrecking my marriage. The pressure on Bob and me was so enormous I'm amazed that we survived it. I went to a support group called Resolve where we all just poured out what was going on, how we felt, and that was the turning point.

'It took me fifteen years in all to accept that I couldn't have a baby. I started at twenty-five and was obsessed the whole time so, yes, of course it was a crisis for me letting go of that obsession, of the longing and the striving which had dominated all those years. I felt so empty, so desperate for a while, but out of that I began to see other ways.'

There tends to be less sympathy for men who reach mid-life not having had children partly because it is often thoughtlessly assumed to be something only women feel really passionately about; or there is the reasoning that men can go on having children far later than women and therefore could change partners and do so.

It is this reasoning that makes Jeremy, a car mechanic who has just turned fifty-five, furious: 'My wife and I have been together since our schooldays and we love each other. I wouldn't just walk out on her because she can't have a kid – how cruel can you get? But we both feel very sad about it and we've been quite depressed in the past few years. It was worst when my brother's wife brought their kids over to see us – we both realized what a lot you miss in life when you can't have a child.'

It is a different kind of distress that Gordon Mann, in his

mid-forties, goes through. He is impotent and his long-term girlfriend left him several years ago because she wanted a child. He says: 'It shattered my confidence and I felt very hurt. I don't want to risk that again. I always imagined I would have children, I very much wanted them, and there is something dreadfully lonely and hopeless about not being able to build a new generation. But I realize it's up to me to come to terms with this and make something different of my life.'

The situation is very different, of course, for those who have chosen not to have children and, having remained clear that this was a right choice, will probably not feel grief or regret. Indeed Imogen Scott, a forty-eight-year-old accountant believes she is likely to suffer less critical feelings than friends coping with empty nests. She says: 'The reason we did not want children is that we enjoy each other's company very much; we have always been very keen on walking and diving and climbing mountains – the kind of thing which would have had to stop for quite a while if we'd had kids and we decided we didn't want to make that sacrifice. I used sometimes to feel quite out of it when friends were all talking about their children, but of course now our life has a pattern, a shape which will not be interrupted unless one of us decides we want a radical change of life. In some ways I think the childless who feel good about it may be the winners at mid-life.'

There is some ambivalence for Leanne George, a journalist and novelist who is on her own and who realized, at forty-four, that she was not going to have children. But she is very clear she must take responsibility for a 'choice' she feels she made. 'I realized I had never made an irrevocable decision and I never had that complete certainty, as some women do, that I didn't want children, but turning that around I never wanted a child enough to make the sacrifices which would have been necessary. I do believe that if you decide not to have children, one of the things you are doing is saying that you want to put creativity and energy into something else.

'In fact I did get pregnant in my thirties and I realized that this might well be my last opportunity, but even then I was quite clear I didn't want the child, and so I had an abortion. I am not faced with the "What have I achieved with my life?" questions. I think I have achieved a considerable amount and that there's plenty more that I can achieve. I feel good about my life. It's stimulating, it's within my grasp to make it what I want, I feel, and that might well not have been so if I had had a child. Indeed right now I feel very strongly that I want to write fiction. It's to do with an unleashing of creativity. I've just finished my first novel and that, to me, IS my baby. So far from flying the nest at mid-life it's being born at this time.'

While women's deepest pain and sense of loss and failure is very often focused in some area of their emotional life, it is observed over and over, how often work and achievement are the focus of men's mid-life crises. Yet this picture is shifting as women make careers in the outside world and invest as much as men do in their working lives. In these circumstances we can see that the time dedicated to emotions and private life frequently shrinks as women's energies go into the competitive and demanding business of building their careers. It seems logical, then, that the issues men face as a result of this will, increasingly, be faced by women too.

Patrick Lindesay, a forty-eight-year-old doctor working near Washington DC, has seen his marriage collapse with angry accusations from his wife that he did not spend enough time with his family. Unfair though this seems when he contemplates the expensive lifestyle his wife aspired to and the work needed to earn enough money, he is nevertheless honest enough to recognize how thoroughly his sense of self is measured by work progress: 'I find myself having the classic thoughts of what have I achieved? Has it been worthwhile? I got very absorbed in my work, became the much admired doctor here, member of the executive committee, kingpin of the area office and that drew me away from the family and seemed important enough that I suppose I justified it.

'Now I see much more clearly that I could have made choices and that my priorities were crazy if I wanted a home life. It's been a very black time and sometimes I've wondered how I would hold together. I can remember one occasion after my wife had moved out with the kids, I was sitting in the cafeteria at the hospital and one of the psychiatrists who I often had breakfast with said: "How are you?" and I answered, as one does: "I'm fine," and he said: "For real, or just I'm fine?" and that just choked me up . . . I was in tears.'

The sense of loss may be less clear-cut than in the case of this doctor. Men who invest the best of their time and emotional energy in work expect that investment to bring them rewards. So when as life moves on through the middle time, and the feelings that the material rewards – promotion, a place in the hierarchy – seem not to add up, men are despondent, angry, betrayed and helpless in knowing how to help themselves. The emptiness inside as they strive, often yet harder, in the external world, becomes increasingly critical.

Paul Buchanan, teacher at a London school, is married with five children, and, during his summer holidays, is regularly invited on foreign study trips. It is, he acknowledges with a wry smile, 'a highly enviable and rather successful life when you look at it dispassionately'. But as he reached forty, there was little dispassion in the way he was viewing his life. He explains: 'I just wanted more than anything to hang on to being young, to know I could go on being young. Forty felt like a landmark time, a time by which I should have achieved what I wanted and to feel that was good enough. You know, one has degrees and further degrees and all these achievements written down on paper but that all felt fairly superficial because I didn't seem to know who I was and I am sure that was part of the crisis I had.

'Nothing I said to myself made me feel that I had lived my life well enough. I just felt that things were passing me by. The sensation was of a boat going somewhere with everybody who I felt had done well on it, but I was left on the shore. It was a very powerful feeling indeed and because of it I was pushing myself, driving myself harder and harder all the time. If I look back I can see that sheer exhaustion with the long hours and the pressing demands of the teenage kids who were in my charge, meant I couldn't take a breathing space or stand back and look at my feelings.

'Then a child in my department committed suicide and it was the worst shock, an appalling tragedy and I felt terribly responsible. It seemed to me that if I had been a better housemaster it wouldn't have happened. It was certainly a trigger which, I think looking back, unleashed all the unhappiness, stress, discontent and anger I was feeling. I'm a person who likes being in control and this was the absolute demonstration that I wasn't in control. And that I suppose is the thing about the mid-life crisis: it shows you that you can't hold everything together and make things the way you want them. You have to go into the abyss and see how to re-construct yourself at the end.'

There is a particular kind of soul-destruction for the person whose work has been a commitment, a passion, a religion, who has worked with an absolute belief in what they are doing, and then finds that it is no longer valued. This is how it was for the talented photographer Don McCullin who had brought to public consciousness some of the very worst atrocities committed against people caught up in wars, living under oppressive regimes, without a voice of their own. He was working for the *Sunday Times* which was moving increasingly towards what he describes in his autobiography, *Unreasonable Behaviour*, as 'leisure and lifestyles'. He found there was less and less interest in the pictures he risked life and personal equilibrium to create. He voiced his disenchantment in an interview with *Granta* magazine and found himself, shortly afterwards, summoned to a meeting with *Sunday Times* editor Andrew Neil. McCullin describes a shabby encounter in which it was 'suggested' that he leave and so, he says: 'I walked out for good from the paper I had served for eighteen years. I went out into a chilly and uncertain world, a middle-aged out-of-work photo-journalist without any prospects.'

For a man used to activity, urgency and an identity fed by the work he did, the world suddenly looked a dismal place. McCullin says: 'Bleak times lay ahead. I tried to meet them with a semblance of the surface confidence which had carried me through dangerous times before. Inside I was a man losing his identity. My whole training had been to look out, to scan the horizon for new stories to tell. Suddenly I was forced to look inwards. In there lurked old darkness and a new guilt from my marriage break-up.' It was a time of utter desolation: 'I was lurking around the flat in Notting Hill . . . I had no commitment. I was lonely. I was hard-up.'

There is a parallel between the empty-nest syndrome and that which men experience when the structure and requirement imposed on them by work disappears. After years with a clear focus, a sense of purpose in life, they must face a void they may have no idea how to fill and of course it is far harder during the times when they feel panicky and uncertain about the world to devise constructive plans and feel optimistic about an uncharted future.

To leave work because retirement age has been reached or because a contract has ended may be bad enough, but it is far harder when we are made redundant or when promotion is refused so that we have to recognize we are no longer valued highly. Realizing that cherished goals will probably never be achieved may be extremely hard to accept. Deidre Sanders, the *Sun* newspaper's agony aunt is confronted with the painful emotional and sexual repercussions of this mid-life sense of failure, day after day: 'There's a lot of coming to terms with disappointment, or dealing with the threat of work ending. Men are experiencing it but the women come to me because they don't know why their men have suddenly gone off them. I have to explain that what is happening is not about them but about their partners trying to find a way to deal with their distress. But of course men often blame the people around them for what feels wrong or they may leave home, go off with another woman – all the things we know so well – in their search for an escape from terrible feelings. That can be extremely hard on a partner. But she needs to try to understand that she is not to blame, because feeling she should have been able to make everything all right is a kind of torture. Of course being supportive, understanding and kind if a man is suffering because he has been made redundant, can't get work, is facing retirement, is something a partner *can* do, but in the end he has to be the one to work out how to go forward.'

Working with men in the Silicon Valley area of California psychotherapist Kenne Zugman has watched the impact on middle-aged men of the high-pressure, high-turnover world. He says: 'The men I see have lived their lives driven by the desire to be somewhere above mid-line in the pecking order. The drive for success, for completion, for living out the prescription of society which means you should keep advancing in your career, is what they see as normal. Then something happens, a trigger, which makes them realize that they are on a path to personal destruction. It may be a shake-up or merger at work which makes them feel very vulnerable or may throw them out of a job; it may be children leaving home and the realization that they have very little communication in their relationship, it may be the death of a parent . . . whatever it is, something happens that unleashes a whole lot of feelings they cannot cope with.'

What strikes him is how intensely men do feel once this happens and how little place there is for this: 'They radiate feelings and in this culture there's no avenue for expression, no permission, no support, no acknowledgement. Men, they have been taught, don't feel – that's what women do. It is an incredible insult to man's deeper poetic soul. And men's experience is to be moved away from a sense of community into a sense of competitiveness if not combativeness. So men hit mid-life not knowing how to locate the cause of their despair and sense of hopelessness. A lot of my work is about tapping that so they don't feel they have to walk out on their lives.'

But there is the flipside to this; the situation where a person – and it is most often men – sees the prospect of continuing in the same work for the rest of their working life, an unbearable prospect. David Smallacombe, director of the Kensington Consultation Centre regularly encounters this: 'For the younger years when people may have been concerned with how far they could take a career, what possibilities may lie ahead, they will be all right even if they don't particularly like what they are doing. But when it becomes the picture of what he or she has done with a whole life, when it is seen as what will have filled most of life, people can feel utterly wretched and trapped. These feelings may be very critical.' Dr Anthony Fry agrees: 'People tend to lay down a blueprint for a career when they are very young and if it does not match what they hoped and planned, but they can see no alternative, people may certainly become very depressed.'

For Vic Seidler, a lecturer and author of books on men and their emotions, critical mid-life feelings were a response to *not* having laid down a blueprint and pursued a career. In his student days he became very committed to left-wing political activities and says:

We had anticipated that we were going to go on with lives that were defined politically but when all that collapsed, when political ideology no longer held, we were left without careers or developed skills. There was a certain edge of bitterness when people went into straight occupations and found that a younger generation were in some way ahead and we didn't get the opportunities we wanted. I'm in my forties and I feel that I've lost out. The causes I invested so much in don't have the same driving force now and there's a general disillusionment with politics, but I don't have a glittering career to make a meaning of my life. I feel angry and upset quite a lot about all this but I do see it as a challenge too. I am now exploring areas of work where the fact that I have some experience of life and psychology will be valued.

It seems clear that we need, as an act of faith, to muster strength, will, humility and courage to deal with what we are facing. Certainly it's no good to protest and parade ourselves as victims who, because we are getting older, can no longer have the centre-stage position. Brenda Polan, a baby-boomer, now in her early fifties, who admits to her own struggles and pain, takes a tough line. She believes that we are generations too used to calling the shots and that we are outraged as well as distressed and disturbed at finding that time prises our hands from life's steering wheel and forces us to realize that we cannot remain in control. She says: 'We have been the biggest, the most vociferous generations, the generations that are deeply complacent because they changed it all. We were needed – the economy couldn't have succeeded without us and we were all able to step into fabulous jobs at a very young age and part of the hideous disillusionment for us now is that we've reached a certain point where the gravy train doesn't seem to go on forever, and we had always assumed it would for us. We're used to having the goodies and the fact that it isn't within our gift to halt the ageing process is very hard.'

Facing the demon of ageing in this light, it may look like all loss and no gain, but, as I will go on to explain, there are gains and rewards to be had from the process of growing up, moving into the next life stage, just as there have been in earlier times. But the gains are the product of having matured and accepted that maturity is right from us and doing this may be a troubled and uncomfortable process. So it is that, in this chapter I have attempted to look at how critical times and actual crises which may occur in mid-life have a purpose which, far from being negative is, in fact, an important part of our ongoing development, a route to psychological well-being in later life. Whether this is how it works out depends, to a considerable extent, on how we deal with our critical times.

We may need guidance in negotiating the mid-life period, the bridge between our life as youngers and the one we go on to lead as elders. How we make the transition is something we have to work out individually, but we may benefit from looking at the ways other people feel they have done so. We can consider the kinds of help and support which others have drawn on and found helpful. Perhaps we can listen to David Lyons who says he struggled every which way to avoid acknowledging that he was ageing and must learn to grow in himself, and who feels he only moved forward when he looked the demon in the eye and told it he would not be beaten.

Look the Demon in the Eye

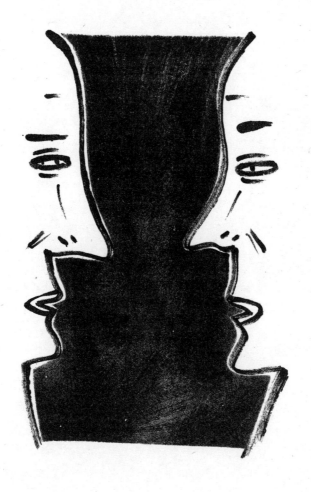

But I know that I shall move. The door will
open slowly and I shall see what there is behind the door.
It is the future. The door to the future will open. Slowly.
Unrelentingly. I am on the threshold.
SIMONE DE BEAUVOIR, *The Woman Destroyed*

Lιfe, observed the writer Alan Bennett, playing a vapid but well-meaning vicar in *Beyond the Fringe*, is rather like opening a tin of sardines. We are all of us looking for the key. Mid-life is a time when we may feel that we should at least have found it. After all, it is at this life-stage, when we have made our way through the years that, in our society, contain the major goals and challenges laid out for us, that we may, quite reasonably, imagine ourselves coming to a moment of assessment, a moment when we may reflect on what has been and process it into something to hold on to – a psychic souvenir pack. So we regard rolling back the lid on life's sardine can as the time to survey our achievements, what we have learned from successes and failures, the things we have done that we feel pleased about and those we squirm to remember, the good, the bad and the ugly. We anticipate it as a time of summation, in which we acknowledge who and what we are, and then, with maturity as the reward for the years lived, we will be ready to make our way to the next stage.

It is a beguiling idea, reassuring in its symmetry, and so long as we are searching for the key, believing we are getting somewhere, anticipating how good the sardines will taste when we have overcome the challenge and peeled back the lid, this notion of how we will make sense of mid-life holds. But then we find the key and open the tin only to find that we've been cheated – the fish is not what we expected, it doesn't taste the way we wanted, it doesn't nourish us as we hoped.

Things are no longer in order, and faith and optimism give way to disillusion and confusion.

The scene is set then for critical times, and my aim in the previous chapter was to look at how they may manifest themselves, how we may feel when they do, what they may be about. In this chapter I am setting out to explore where the experience of critical times may take us. I am looking to find a reason in what can seem random and meaningless upheaval and distress, making a mockery of our belief that we have matured and strengthened through the years, that we are equipped to live life in a more self-assured and tranquil way than many of us achieved in earlier years. What a farce the chirrupy cry of Ogden Nash, 'Middle-age is merry, And I love to live it,' can seem: we put much of our energy and conviction into trying to find ways of avoiding facing up to the message of the distress. Jung expressed well the urgent need we may feel *not* to look at the idea that it is perhaps a time at which we need to question our value system, to be prepared to make alterations for the next part of our journey:

Every one of us gladly turns away from his problems; if possible, they must not be mentioned, or, better still, their existence is denied. We choose to have certainties and no doubts – results and no experiments – without even seeing that certainties can arise only through doubt, and results through experiment. The artful denial of a problem will not produce conviction; on the contrary, a wider and higher consciousness is called for to give us the certainty and clarity we need.

Yet I have become convinced by what I have learned from working on this book, from talking to people with very different attitudes to life, from reading texts by those who range in their approaches from the spiritual and philosophical to the scientific and from my own experience of going into a deep, dark place for a while and finding, extraordinarily, that something valuable has come from what I was forced to grasp: that we do indeed cheat, and possibly harm, ourselves if we will not accept and learn from our mid-life critical times. Our task, I believe, is to see these as a route (a circuitous one, perhaps) that, if we will take it, enables us to gain knowledge and understanding that will guide us on the next part of our journey, a route that can lead us to a greater understanding of our own – human – dimension.

We may not choose to go through critical times, yet it is remarkable how many people echo the sentiments of Bonnie Norton, who describes in the previous chapter getting into an affair which ended, leaving her 'overwhelmed with an immovable pain, as though I were disintegrating', but who, once she had come through that pain, says emphatically that she emerged with a feeling of confidence she had not had before, a sense of knowing herself better than before and the knowledge of strengths which could now be called upon. She talked of a very tangible ability she had been forced to acquire in order to cope with emotional pain – something she sees as a valuable part of her armoury for life ahead.

William, who began drinking a great deal in his early forties to dull what he described as the 'grey, grey sense of futility inside me', retreated farther and farther from his wife, blaming her, he says, for not being able to make the world feel good, for the fact that he thought life was finished for him. For eighteen months he felt as though everything was slipping away from him. It was when he overheard a friend telling his wife that he was a man who had the sense of having died that he realized his condition was serious and that he must stop trying to blot out what was happening. He says: 'I didn't know how to do that, but what happened was that I went away. I took time off work and just went away by myself, walking in Scotland. I stayed in crofters' cottages, and I went through this curious process of hearing myself think. At first it was like a babble of all the things I felt were wrong with life, my reasons for being angry, for drinking – something I didn't do at all during this time. Then after about three days that all calmed down, and I began to be filled with a feeling of being calm and that life was a good place. I began to feel quite optimistic, although not about anything in particular, and when I got home I felt that by going into a quiet space, by daring to let myself feel, I felt good. Of course, it wasn't all easy going home, and life wasn't magically transformed, but I stopped feeling I had to drink so much, and I could see much more clearly that my wife was not the problem in my life. Just recognizing those things enabled me to feel better and stronger.'

These are just two stories among many that tell us about a kind of progress, something that Peter Hildebrand, who led workshops on the second half of life, refers to when he talks of recent evidence which suggests that a developmental process takes place in us all in later adulthood, when the events that make up a mid-life critical time disrupt 'previously adaptive systems with challenges which lead to conflict, tension and potentially the evolution of new and more satisfactory solutions, leading to changes in the way we think about ourselves and our relationships to others'.

There is, then, a strong, muscular body of conviction to suggest that, perverse as this may seem, we have reason to welcome our critical times and view them as opportunities for worthwhile change. My aim is to explore these, the possible gains from the disappointment of the unsatisfactory sardines. But we need, too, to understand that the process is not a simple, fast-fix formula, even though there are certainly people who find they have got themselves over their humps in a short space of time. Rather, we would do well to regard the hard times as periods of learning, which, like others, take time and a way of staying with the learning. This point is well expressed in the words of psychotherapist Diana Glassner, whose clients include those grappling with mid-life and those who have moved some way on from it. She says: 'We tend to see mid-life as being like a precipice and think we will just tilt over into old age, but in fact it's a gradual process leading there, and I believe we have to have faith that we can adjust and accept as we go along and that it won't match up to our terrible imaginings.'

We hear something of that in the way actress Sheila Hancock construes what was a time of physical and psychological crisis for her, and it is striking how often a fatal threat at mid-life acts as a catalyst, making us realize that we do not want to waste any more time on living in an unsatisfactory, compromised way. We see the importance of changing course, of looking at our own needs and learning to consider what is necessary for us if we are to go on growing as we age. It is not selfishness but quite legitimate recognition that we want something more, in terms of spiritual and emotional satisfaction, than has been possible hitherto. Actress Sheila Hancock contracted cancer and felt she must leave her actor husband John Thaw because 'our marriage was going through a dodgy period,' from which we may extrapolate that, as happens with so many couples in the middle years, the pattern and emotional framework which had carried them through the earlier years no longer seemed an adequate framework for the time ahead. Hancock explained in an interview with writer Deborah Moss: 'I needed to be alone. I had always known what John wanted. And what the children wanted. And what the National [Theatre] wanted. But not what I wanted. All my life I had leaned on men. First my father. Then my first husband. Then John. I had known myself only as reflections of them. Now I needed to be me.' She does not elaborate on what she went through during the time of separation, but it was, clearly, an important part of moving towards being a person who seems to have new perceptions and plenty of spirit for what lies ahead. She explains what appears to her the central point of the growth she has experienced: 'The separation [from John] made us both much less reliant on each other. We both now know we can survive on our own, which seems healthier and better somehow.'

Hancock is typical of women in framing her discontent around her emotional life; it is less often so clearly a bid for emotional survival in men. Yet the situation of Graham Hall, a forty-nine-year-old joiner, although different, shows too a recognition of his emotional needs surfacing that he felt was forced upon him. He had been at loggerheads with his brother since his twenties and, he says: 'Through the years I justified my anger with him. I persuaded other people to agree with me and blocked out the sadness I knew was there at having effectively lost Joe, my brother. Then – I remember the day – I was in my middle forties when I heard that Joe was getting married. I felt as though I wanted to cry – howl, really. I couldn't understand why, and as the weeks went by I was just very depressed. I was living on my own because I'd never got married and normally that had been fine, but now it didn't feel at all fine. In the end I was so low I told a good friend, a woman I've known for years, how down I felt, mentioning that it had started when I heard about Joe's wedding. This friend got me to talk about my relationship with Joe when we were kids – we were really close then – and all sorts of stuff came up: the holidays we'd had as teenagers, how he had doted on me . . . all sorts of stuff. By the end I was full of all these memories, and I kept trying to stop myself crying.

'My friend didn't say much, but when we were parting she told me I should try to make things up with Joe. My first reaction was to say, "Stuff that." But I kept thinking about Joe and realizing how much I wanted to see him again. I found it very hard to think about making the first advance, but I did – I wrote a rather cautious letter congratulating him on his marriage and saying I was sorry we'd lost touch. The day he got it he rang, and we arranged to meet. It was sticky at first, but I just felt so pleased to see him that I think it showed, and I didn't feel any anger any more. We talked a bit about what we'd been doing, but then it got on to times past because I mentioned I'd been thinking about that. By the end we were hugging each other. It was like a miracle. The depression lifted and I saw a life full of times ahead with my brother and his wife, who was very warm and welcoming.'

Graham is convinced that what happened had a lot to do with being at mid-life. The news of Joe's wedding might not have changed anything much in reality, as they had been separated so long, but symbolically it felt like a definitive move. He explains: 'I felt that Joe was becoming part of a new family and that I was left abandoned. But, of course, I didn't see that I felt upset at the idea that he really would be lost to me. Instead I told myself he was a fool, that the woman was probably a bitch – all sorts of stuff I'm ashamed to admit now. But underneath I felt terribly bleak and as though I was full of a dark fog. I think it is extraordinarily lucky that I talked to my friend, and she somehow made it possible for me to break through my angry façade, because I think otherwise I'd have just got more and more bitter and miserable as I got older. I am at an age when I think our roots, the people who are part of our history, matter very much, and I feel so glad that the future looks better now with the knowledge that I have Joe back in my life.'

What we learn from the life events in our maturer years is often quite different from what we learned in the first half of our lives, but the way we deal with that learning is also different. It is up to us to let go of some of our coping mechanisms, patterns of behaviour, fixed beliefs, fear of losing face and identity. We need to do this, Jung believed, as a way of opening up a new innocence, a childlike willingness to learn afresh, if we are to find a way to be at peace with our inner feelings and yearnings, rather than trying, as we so often do, to push away anything uncomfortable. Rosalind Milton, who has been through a considerable crisis, as we shall see later on, feels she has emerged with new understanding. She describes how essential it was to stop trying to escape from what was going on inside her by keeping hectically busy, to be brave enough to risk the pain that might be there and 'feel the feelings'. David Lyons sees mid-life as the time when we are full of anxiety and uncertainty, and he suggests we need to 'look the demon in the eye and stay put, absorbing its stare and understanding what it means rather than running scared'.

In talking to people, who are often reluctant to admit that they have floundered and felt helplessly stuck, I have been struck by this imagery and by their sense of the disintegration of what had seemed their essential self, how close it feels to the way Yeats describes the breakdown of structure in 'The Second Coming':

> Things fall apart; the centre cannot hold;
> Mere anarchy is loosed upon the world,
> The blood-dimmed tide is loosed, and everywhere
> The ceremony of innocence is drowned . . .

If we can understand the universality of this feeling, it may help us to listen to, rather than deride (as all too often happens in our determinedly coping culture), those people who believe they have gained an understanding of themselves and the human condition through their struggles. Instead, as Terri Apter notes in *Secret Paths*, her exploration of women in what she argues is a new mid-life because of the changes which have occurred in women's lives this past half century, women (and, I would say, men too) all too easily deny the 'psychological descent' that has so often taken place before they have become, as a butterfly emerging from a chrysalis, a renewed and enlarged person. Apter cites Gloria Steinem who is indeed an impressive woman, whom years of heading up feminism with less stridency and more wit than many of her sisters appear to have moulded into something pretty special as she enters her sixties. But Apter points to how Steinem, from her present vantage point, 'looks askance at the jumble of her younger adult self, seeing much of her past self as shallow or misguided or off-center, without appreciating how this shifting perspective was a developmental process'. She takes Gail Sheehy, author of a number of life-stage books, to task too for the way in which, in *The Silent Passage*, she 'notes, but only in passing, the turmoil women in their forties suffer. She uses this turmoil as a point of comparison, to show how much better off women are once they pass fifty; she fails to see that it is an essential step toward that special phase of women's maturity she so eloquently embraces.'

In this chapter, which is intended as a sequel to the previous one, my intention is to look at how, along with finding our own, private ways of accepting and developing, we may also do well to seek help and guidance when going through our critical times. Although sometimes, as in the stories above, people find ways by themselves or within their own circle, this does not always happen.

It is not easy to acknowledge to oneself, let alone admit publicly, to a mid-life crisis. Who will willingly concede such human frailty in a culture where, from childhood, we are taught that being on top, in control, number one, is the most important thing? How, after decades of conforming to such an ethos, can we suddenly say, 'Excuse me, I have no conviction about anything any more. Being a success at work doesn't feel that marvellous any longer. My partner and I seem to live on separate tracks these days, and all I really want to do is go and live in an ashram in India or take up scuba diving in the Red Sea'?

Not many of us dare. Keeping quiet about feelings of weakness or failing conviction is the way we have learned to survive. 'Shut up, shut down and SMILE' is one message we beam to our inner selves when things feel critical; the other is 'Quick, find a diversion, a fast fix, so I don't have to live with these uncomfortable feelings.' Sheila Kitzinger, in discussing Western societies' attitudes, points out that we will go to almost any lengths to blot out pain, even when it is enabling us to understand something as profound as birth. We no longer believe there is a place for pain: if we experience physical discomfort, we reach for the analgesics; if the pain is psychic, we pop Prozac. Dr Fry likens our quest to eliminate imperfection to medical science's quest for the bionic heart. He says: 'We have reached a stage where technology can replace the bits of the body which pack up so that we can go on functioning. On one level that may be marvellous, but what it also tells us is that we should be able to function no matter what breakdown is going on. When people reach middle age and have to face the fact that the body becomes more frail and our dreams have to be moderated, they cannot pause and acknowledge that this is a time to assess who they are and where they are. Rather they see a world where not being in perfect nick and able to replicate younger generations makes you a write-off.'

In such a culture it is realistic to assume that the person who tells the boss at work that they are in turmoil and can't make sense of life is more likely to be shown the door than offered a shoulder to cry on. When marriages break up in mid-life there is a strong climate of condemnation, a sense that we have failed rather than that we need support and sympathy. And the man who couples up with a much younger woman in what may well be a desperate but inchoate attempt to offset fears about ageing can expect every kind of reproof. If you reach for the bottle in the hope that it will blot out the bad feelings, rather than daring to voice them, this will more likely be judged as the first step on the downhill slope than a cry for help. The same conclusion is drawn by Nancy Mayer, author of a study of men at mid-life, who writes: 'The man who craves renewal at mid-life cannot count on much help from society. For the most part he will have to work through the crisis period alone, and to do so he will have to struggle to overcome in himself many of the beliefs he shares with the culture in which he lives.'

Yet it is a universal struggle and one with which people from every walk of life and social background grapple. Some do it entirely alone, attempting to avoid acknowledging what is going on; others turn to sympathetic friends, as Graham did, and find great comfort in being heard as they struggle to explain the inexplicable and, through doing this, come to a *rapprochement* with themselves. Others set themselves new challenges to overcome a sense of futility, or enter into some therapeutic, spiritual or psychological process in order to learn a new way of living in the world. The ways people choose to try to work through the mid-life critical times are as different as the individuals' personalities and circumstances, but for many the toughest part is a sense of isolation, of being alone in finding that their centre doesn't seem to be holding any longer and of not understanding what is going on or how it may be possible to pull through.

Ken Wilkie now has a long-term relationship and two children with the woman he almost lost through his inability to realize that forever trying to keep all his options open was not possible. He was just into his forties, and he believes that an unresolved relationship with his mother – which meant that, through earlier years, he had sought a maternal figure in his relationships, then backed off when the women wanted a more equal commitment – had much to do with the fact that he remained emotionally immature at mid-life. Looking back on all this, he recognizes, with relief, the path that his deep despair led him down.

Ken says: 'I was having an affair with Laura, wanting her and knowing I was risking losing her because I couldn't give up the other woman I had been with for years. I didn't feel I could make a commitment to either of them, and it was driving us all slightly mad. Laura then met somebody else, and it hit me that I could not be sure she would be there for me, and I went into panic and terror. None of the apparent freedom, the keeping my options open, that I'd so wanted to hang on to seemed worth anything. There was nothing anybody could say to help because there was every possibility Laura would decide to live with this other man. I knew I had to do something to sort myself out, and there seemed no way, if I went on as I was, to get clarity of mind. I stopped seeing both women. I felt totally alone, absolutely stripped down and just desperate with misery. It was at this time that my dog died, and that felt like the biggest thing in the world. I became quite ill and felt as though I were disintegrating. I don't remember ever feeling so alone, so utterly, deeply in the bowels of life and so unable to sort things out. The irony was that I was editing a publication, looked up to by other people as having status and wisdom, but I had no resources to draw on.

'But I think now that I had to get to that state to be able to grow up, literally to stop wanting to be the kid who has all the goodies. In that state of misery I began to see clearly the value of building something with stability, with the kind of love that is about cherishing someone not just about being on an ego trip. I drew back from the socializing I'd been doing; I walked a lot, talked a lot with friends and spent a lot of time on my own. It took that to make me realize that being quiet and in my own company felt okay – good, in fact. But there was a long time of being in a state of just existing in the moment, until Laura decided she was happy to have our relationship. The good thing about having made a commitment at this fairly late stage is that I feel able to look back and see that things weren't so great before, when I seemed to be able to be king of the castle and play the field. It was possible to see what pleasure there is in building up a home together, pottering in the garden with my kids, creating a small but significant world. I began to feel much calmer and more settled, and I now have a vision of a life with Laura, growing older together and enjoying our children and, in due course, grandchildren.'

What we learn in listening to the voices here is that things can change without our needing necessarily to make drastic manoeuvres that up-end our lives, throw our history out of the window, or keep us trapped in a damaging false pride. If we accept the thesis of the previous chapter, that the mid-life critical times have a very real developmental purpose, then it may be easier to face the feelings which, like hostile forces, seem to invade us.

Finding a way that she believed had illuminated later life was the experience of Helen Luke, an American writer who, in her eighties, produced five beautiful essays on the theme of old age. In 'Suffering' she asks us to look at the impulse we have to banish pain and psychic discomfort (touched on earlier) at any price, and she states unequivocally what has been said to me many, many times, although in less certain terms: that the only valid cure for the dark, confusing feelings lies in accepting them, acknowledging that things are, at this minute, painful. In doing this, we come to a state in which we are not struggling, and the psyche is able to begin the business of sorting itself out. Luke explains her interpretation of what goes on when we are grappling with our critical times, attempting very often to hold on to all the things that have seemed to make us what we are, to retain the sense of our own importance in the world at a time when we may be feeling diminished by the loss of our young self, by the prospect of becoming an elder in a culture where that has so pejorative a meaning. She suggests:

Nothing whatever has happened to the soul. The roots of all our neuroses lie here, in the conflict between the longing for growth and freedom and our incapacity or refusal to pay the price in suffering of the kind which challenges the supremacy of the ego's demands ... The ego will endure the worst agonies of neurotic misery rather than one moment of consent to the death of even a small part of its demand or its sense of importance.

Something similar is expressed by psychologist Dorothy Rowe, who has seen how, in our attempts to deny and defy the ageing process, we try to find ways to block out reality. But denial may make our dark fears worse, Rowe says. She sees that fear means glimpsing our own insignificance, vulnerability, helplessness, isolation, weakness and fragility, but believes that, however painful this is, it is only by confronting the fear face to face, acknowledging what it is we feel and why, then working to get beyond it, that we can find a way to make things better. To take the other path and try to avoid facing our fear is to risk, she says, annihilating the self that is the core of our being, our self-esteem, the person we must live with. Unresolved fear that leads on to despair stems, at least in part, in the view of the pre-eminent psychoanalyst Erik Erikson (*Childhood and Society*), a man whose own life journey was an endless quest for enlightenment, from our refusal to accept that we must move on in life, that things have to change.

But this does not mean settling for a lesser life: rather, it means accepting a challenge that can lead us to experience and understand things in a new way; it can liberate us from a strait-jacketing value-system; it can prompt us to try new ways of doing things, to embark on schemes we would not have contemplated so long as we were tied up with our early-life personae. The process may not be simple or painless. As we have heard, people experience very real emotional pain when they are struggling to find the route to integrity, and it can be difficult to accept not feeling good in a culture that bombards us with the idea that we should be eternally happy – and if we are not, we should be able to buy something, study something, find a guru or whatever, to lead us to happiness. If we cannot achieve happiness, we are endlessly told, that is our failing.

Yet accepting that we cannot be happy all the time may be far healthier than it feels. This is the view of Dr Michael Scott Peck, whose writings about his own quest for inner peace have made him an international bestseller. In his work Scott Peck has, he says, seen many people making themselves mentally ill by avoiding problems and emotional suffering, and he voices sentiments quite similar to Luke's: 'Some of us will go to quite extraordinary lengths to avoid our problems and the suffering they cause, proceeding far afield from all that is clearly good and sensible in order to try to find an easy way sometimes to the total exclusion of reality. When we avoid the legitimate suffering that results from dealing with problems, we also avoid the growth that problems demand from us.'

But what, we may ask, do Scott Peck and the others mean precisely? Isn't it normal, if life feels out of sync, to look for a solution? Yes, indeed, but the question is: are we looking for a solution that will benefit us, lead us forward with that integrity that Erikson believes is vital to our psychological well-being, or will our 'solution' simply provide a temporary fix? We see every day around us men and women cutting off erstwhile friends or colleagues because they confront them with an unpalatable truth, speak honestly to them, ask that they understand an aspect of their behaviour that is intolerable. It may seem a 'solution' to find new friends with whom we can reinvent ourselves. If our relationships appear to be unsatisfactory, dull places to be, our partner appears to limit who we believe we can be, then the 'solution' may seem to be to find somebody new as a way to escape yet not suffer the pain of aloneness or the realization of what we have done. Of course, as I will move on to later, there are times when having the courage to leave a relationship that has been tried to the limit, and is destructive and damaging, may also be the courageous and difficult thing to do. If our children disappoint us by not matching our expectations, it may seem a 'solution' to disdain them for fear that otherwise we may lose face in front of friends or colleagues. If we recognize that we are afraid of ageing, we may look for a lover or a new clique to join, in a younger age-group, as a way of trying to acquire some chronological credit.

Each of these 'solutions' may seem to have done the trick for a while, but the chances are that they will not banish the internal struggles we were confronting, which consultant psychiatrist Dr Anthony Fry, among many others, believes constitute the unavoidable knowledge of our own entropy. This is not a moral judgement: it is not appropriate for outsiders to assess the decisions people make without knowing who they are or why they make their choices. It is a practical judgement, one based on my own anecdotal evidence and, more substantially, the work of many of those working in different disciplines where human behaviour is analysed.

Through these different voices a similar idea emerges. Each is pointing out that we need to accept and feel what is going on and to try to understand its meaning. Fiona Boswell, a psychotherapist who practises in London, sums up: 'There is such strong denial, such a conviction that these feelings are about nothing serious and have no right to be there, and so people feel angry with themselves for not being able to shake off the feelings ... I see people at mid-life changing relationships or punishing their partners because they cannot just stay with their feelings and try to understand why they may be there. But it is only when they can start looking at what is going on inside them, that feels so unacceptable, that I see them becoming less desperate, calmer, less terrified of what they are feeling and then able to explore more honestly what they want to do.'

It is not surprising that we want a rational explanation for what is going on, and developmentalists who have studied the human psyche at this stage in life believe there *is* a way of understanding. Psychologist Daniel Levinson talks of the imperative to break out of a 'life-structure' in order to create a new direction that will make sense of the time ahead and enable us to begin our journey into the new life-stage as a young elder, embarking on a period of growing up and maturing just as we did at that other crucial life-stage, adolescence. It is a time at which we must let go of our tenure in the youth camp, let that phase of life become a past which we can cherish and refer to with pleasure and fond memories, rather than dreading each passing year because it tells us ever more plainly that we no longer belong to the earlier era. Then we are faced with a new, empty canvas, and the picture on it will be drawn and filled in with the story of our future. It may be difficult to lose the familiar images of time past, but it can also be seen as an opportunity to put away the story of the first part of our life that contains disappointments, failures, the ways we have behaved which shame us, the shabbiness of things we have done, as well as its good and positive features. Writer Ralph Waldo Emerson saw moving on as an adventure from which we return with new awareness:

Be not the slave of your own past,
Plunge deep into the sublime seas,
Dive deep, and swim far
So you shall come back
With self respect
With new power
With an advanced experience,
That shall explain
And overlook the old.

Emerson sees clearly how, in this time that may so easily feel like the death of all we have valued, there is an opportunity for renewal. And so, as we roll up the canvas of the picture of the first half of life, we can celebrate having a new canvas on which we may start something other, a picture of this next stage, which can be excitingly different, an exposition of our personal development, of what we have become in our time. It will be a picture with different themes and perspectives. We can contemplate how to be the kind of person we would wish to be in the future; we can consider, with knowledge and maturity, what picture of us we would like the new canvas to present; and we can think about how to live this new life-stage in a way that will make this fresh presentation possible. Buddhists see clearly the significance of the point at which we stand: 'What you are now is the past; what you will become is the present.'

But many of us will have lived the first part of our lives in industrialized Western societies where we have learned rules and regulations, clear instructions about the way things should and should not be done, from our earliest age, so it is hardly surprising that we long for a strategy for action, a ground plan with a clearly defined course. We seek the reassurance of obstacles and of ways to negotiate them, laid out like a challenge, which, if we apply ourselves, can be overcome. Mihaly Csikzentmihalyi, who runs seminars for business executives in America on how to handle the mid-life crisis, talks of how he sees men flailing at finding that their well-developed skills, all that they have achieved and accumulated, make no difference to the confusion and despair they feel at realizing that the centre is not holding. Psychotherapist Kenne Zugman, working with men in California, including many who work at a very high level in the computer industry in Silicon Valley, sees the same in his clinic. He says: 'They are experiencing what the philosophical American writer Joseph Campbell describes as having put our ladder against the wall, put all our effort into climbing it, then feeling at mid-life that we chose the wrong wall. What I try to help my clients do is to see that it may not be the wrong wall but that they need to find a different position for the ladder. It is around the fifties that I see this the most. It is hard for men who have reached this stage to realize that they may need to be brave enough to let go of a value system which keeps them endlessly striving, struggling to be validated by the outer world, a pay cheque, a job title, how well the kids have done . . . whatever. It's not a question of their necessarily needing to stop being interested in their job or enjoying things they have valued, but rather that they need to relinquish a bit of the power these things have over them so that they can shift the balance of their lives. Perhaps then they can start finding space to develop other aspects of who they are which they have ignored throughout the busy years of climbing the ladder.'

Hearing Zugman, I recognized well what he was saying. He may have been talking about men – and more men than women lead lives on what is, effectively, a monorail throughout their young adulthood – but women do it too, although less often so dedicatedly around work. But we may well construct an image around a number of things which have to be maintained, we believe, for us to feel all right. For years I prided myself on presenting a picture to the world of the woman who managed a demanding freelance career, a large house and two live-wire sons and who had, to all appearances, succeeded in achieving that rare thing, the harmonious and egalitarian relationship with a partner. It felt good when people complimented me on these achievements, and, a bit like a junkie, I needed my dose of external approval. My own self-approval didn't suffice; it wasn't convincing. I needed the currency of approbation from those whom I was striving to impress. There was a high price to pay, although I didn't recognize it at the time, for keeping up this image – because the truth was that my life was not, and is not, a picture of perfection. Like most people's lives, it is a mix of the good, the bad and the mediocre. At times my career seems to ride high; at other times I feel it has plateaued and that, at my stage in life, I should have achieved far more. Sometimes I feel on top of everything, able to juggle kids, work, running my home and having time for friends with ease; at other times there is the sense that I'm living in a food-processor and cannot keep it all going. As for my relationship it is the oldest story in the world – good bits and bad bits, times of tangible pleasure and togetherness and times when I feel we're badly mismatched (and my partner clearly feels the same).

Keeping the image intact meant that I could not admit to feeling not good enough, a failure at times, an empty shell at other times. Looking back, it seems bizarre that in some way I never articulated to myself that there was the deepest fear of rejection and self-loathing if anyone saw behind the stage-set of my act. I couldn't contemplate admitting that I was screaming inside because there was no outlet when the going got tough, when troubles and problems occurred. I did not have the knowledge or the awareness to decipher the messages from my psyche. I didn't link the dark times, when I felt unbearably lonely, with the fact that I was pushing away and refusing to acknowledge negative feelings. It seems to me no coincidence that the structure cracked when I reached mid-life. I had been very much aware, from my early forties, of the feeling that I had had my chances, that everything worth while had passed, that the picture I had painted was fading fast. I found myself one Saturday morning, head down, sobbing on the kitchen table of a close woman friend. I howled over a row I had had with my partner, and how badly I had handled things, and how hopeless it all seemed; I was distraught because one of my sons was being bolshie and difficult; I had submitted an article to a newspaper which I knew was badly thought out and shoddily written, and I was in torment over that. It was as though my entire house of cards had collapsed, and suddenly I was admitting it because I couldn't do anything else.

It was the best thing that could have happened. By admitting that I was not capable of running everything well enough to be an object of admiration, envy even, I created a space for my friend to come in and talk me through what was going on. She asked why it mattered to me so much to appear to be a kind of super-woman. Why was I afraid to be ordinary? she asked. They were important questions, which in due course I explored with a therapist and found myself embarked on a quite thrilling exploration. That exploration enabled me to let the perfect image go, to be braver and more daring in my relationships with other people. What happened also allowed my friend, when in due course she had problems, to come to me – something she had never done before because, I suspect, nobody wants to talk to someone who appears to cope super-well. I realized that acknowledging being as ordinary and as imperfect as anyone else felt fine. It was a wonderful liberation. From that time on I felt able to use my own experiences when people came to me with their difficulties; it led me to far greater understanding and, I like to think, empathy with others. Certainly my friendships became closer, and I became much tougher about what I wanted from my relationship with my partner which, far from wreaking havoc, strengthened what we have. Out of all this came a new confidence and a sense of pleasure at what I may now be able to go forward and experience.

I have found myself turning, often, to Jung while thinking about these themes. As the founder of Analytical Psychology, he made it his task to explore what universal experiences there are, while working always to achieve and understand an ever greater spiritual dimension to his own existence, and I believe he has much of worth to tell us. He was convinced that, if we can understand the rewards of learning to find support and succour for ourselves from within, we can be more fulfilled and contented than if we rely endlessly on the approval the outside world gives (with its flipside, the suffering when that approval is withheld or when there is disapproval). Jung believed, as other explorers of the psyche do, that through doing this we experience a kind of growth and strengthening at the core that is something other than the way in which we grow in the first part of life. He expressed it this way: 'The greatest potential for growth and self-realization exists in the second half of life.'

More comforting than the prospect of the tough process of growing through pain is to believe that the feelings can be thrown off, dumped and left. Penny Valentine, fifty, observes: 'I have this picture of putting all the emotional baggage I feel I've been lugging around for years into a black plastic sack and dumping it in the corner of a room then walking away – carefree. But, of course, I know that bag would find a way to join me because what is going on is the stuff which has never been dealt with properly from long ago. Mid-life has thrown it up because I'm scared of what I'm going to do when I've finished being a mother in a few years.'

Brian Larkston, too, surveys fifty-four years and analyses with a certain perceptiveness how he has 'spent most of my adult life protecting myself from getting hurt. I've done it particularly in my relationships with women. I've played at intimacy but never let it get too close to me because I cannot bear the idea of being rejected. I've always made sure I was the person who broke relationships off rather than letting my partners do it, and I've been quite brutal rather than risk letting a woman feel she had touched me deeply. I'm in a relationship now, living with a woman and her two children, but it's the same thing: I feel detached, and she suffers because of that, and I would like to find a way of breaking through what has been called commitment phobia. Someone suggested therapy, but I found myself saying, "I don't want to risk being unravelled" – and that's just it. I fear everything will get into chaos and there'll be no way of making sense of myself again if I risk looking at why I'm the way I am. But I'm not happy with it – it's a lonely way to be and I am frightened of getting old in this state.'

But even if we can grasp that there is no straightforward way of dealing with these feelings, the question remains: what to do? The unconscious does not send us instructions. How, when grappling with a heart of darkness, do we know which way to go, how to make sense of what the disruptive internal voice is urging? It is not a new dilemma: Dante confronted his mid-life crisis six hundred years ago. In his beautiful allegorical discourse *Divina Commedia* he describes the sense of being lost, frightened with no sense of guidance: 'In the middle of the journey of life . . . I found myself inside a dark forest, for the right way I had completely lost.' He tells of the dangers, appearing as wild animals, representing ambition, lust and greed, that might destroy him and how, by way of rescue, the ghost of the poet Virgil appears and offers to show him the way out of the forest – but that way leads through Hell, and that is the path Dante must take.

Psychologist Elizabeth Wilde McCormick, who has written about mid-life crisis, says: 'We may be literally forced by the unconscious into a new phase that at the beginning we really do not understand . . . We are challenged to find meaning: what has my life been about so far? What do I want to keep? The crises we find in ourselves do not immediately let us know this is what our struggle is about.'

That was certainly true for Australian Terry Neale, forty-five. He had been teaching in schools for fifteen years, moving often in pursuit of promotion, behaving in a way he knew would please the father who had always pushed himself and was proud of his work ethic. One day Terry found himself sitting at a classroom desk, tears falling through the hands he had stretched over his face. He went into the Principal and said he was leaving. He consulted a psychiatrist, terrified that he was going mad. He says: 'I realized through him that I had had to make myself ill before I could allow myself to risk breaking out of the trap I felt I was in.'

Nor did Rosalind Milton, a single mother of a daughter who has just turned fifty, whose creative, humanitarian work had played a vital role in her life, understand what her crisis was about when she found herself literally, as she believed, struggling for life. She traces the beginning of her awareness of things being wrong to when her office reorganized and she found herself working for a new boss, under whom she began to feel diminished and undermined. As she became less and less able to do the job as she wished, despair began to set in. It took her more than a year to summon up the courage to leave the job, and she says, reflecting: 'I had structured my life pretty rigorously, as my way of keeping the show on the road for me and my child. The structures kept our lives together, but they were a prison, too. In that office situation the heart went out of me and my work, so only the structures were left. And that was deadly. I know now that I was carrying a lot of stuff from the past that I had never faced or resolved – a lot of pain. The structures cut me off and protected me from all that. But they also trapped me in it and stopped me moving forward.

'At work I tried to get through what I told myself was just a bad patch. But it went deep. This boss, a woman, was unpleasant in the way only women can be to each other. Even so long afterwards I felt she had destroyed something in me. I fought to keep going, but by the end there was no choice or decision to make. I just wanted to *stop*. My instinct told me to get out to save my life.

'So I did. I think that act did save me. But it was also a kind of death. And in this period – about three years – the whole of my old life died. Not just that job, but almost every aspect of my existence ended or changed. It was frightening. I didn't know how I would replace either the structures or the income that came with my work. But I felt that I had to let those structures fall away to find my own centre – to find if I *had* a centre.'

After she had made the break from her old life, Rosalind became ill and faced the diagnosis and treatment of cancer, and she believes this was a physical manifestation of the same process. She explains: 'I now see everything that happened as a kind of metaphor. I think that if we deny or bury our past pain, it comes up to meet us in our present lives, like some monster we've kept hidden in a dungeon. We can't run away from it for ever; the longer we do, the bigger it will grow. We have to face it.' An analysis, a returning to roots, has come through the time she has spent on her own, very quietly, letting the spirit rest and heal, rather as her body had to do after her operation, and recuperate from the trauma it had been through.

Listening to Rosalind talking now, three years since she made the decision to leave her job, I am struck by the calm in her but also the humanity, the way she listens to *my* preoccupations, the generosity with which she gives time to think about what I am saying. I am aware that she seems to have reached an acceptance of herself and her life which is so very different from the way she was when caught in her distressing impasse: fraught, nervy, seeming to need to keep the world at bay in case it overloaded her life and tipped her into chaos. She explains: 'I think my monster grew from a very old, early feeling that I was not only unloved but unlovable – that there was no love for me and there never would be any love for me. And if you're not loved, as a tiny child, you're not quite there. You're nothing. At heart I felt I didn't really exist. And I didn't really want to exist.'

Rosalind spent months living very simply in her flat: reading, writing, thinking, 'just being', coming to face the inner emptiness and the loss of her professional identity. During this time all kinds of memories, feelings and fragments of experience surfaced: annihilating sadnesses from childhood, the betrayal and rejection by her child's father, the bullying of her former boss. There were many small, unexpected pleasures, too: 'A cup of tea, a hot bath, a letter, a wonderful book, a meeting with a friend'. Therapy helped; so did prayer. 'Even the cancer had a positive aspect – it felt like my body's way of clearing the damage from the past.'

She now looks back on this period as a time of healing and transformation. 'It allowed me to feel my feelings, to under-stand my life better, to accept the past and let it go. It's cleared a lot of old stuff and created a space in which I can build a new life and faith in myself. I'm not saying that I'm now a totally strong, brand-new person. I still feel anger, fear, sad-ness, at times. But I feel different, too. My ambivalence about life has gone. I really *want* to live now and to live in a new way.'

We process our mid-life feelings in different ways and with different degrees of intensity, but for some of us the sense of being broken down, of seeing no simple way to make things hold together, is what we must accept if we are to find a new way of being. In his poem 'The Phoenix' D. H. Lawrence expresses precisely how ego's annihilation may be the route to growing in a new way:

> Are you willing to be sponged out, erased, cancelled,
> made nothing?
> Are you willing to be made nothing?
> dipped into oblivion?
>
> If not, you will never really change.

Laurence Hughes, whose young life as one of a large working-class Irish family did not bring him much into contact with the contemplative, has turned that way as he reaches his fifties. As a result of a near breakdown, caused by stress at work and alcohol, he turned to men's groups for support and help. He talks of being, at this time, in the midst of terrible bleakness and believes there was no effective way to escape feeling what was going on. He describes how this was for him: 'I was planning a holiday for myself and the children. I was immensely busy at work, and I was aware that everything going on inside me was on the back burner. Then I got on the boat to France for the holiday, and suddenly the pressure was off. I was flooded with all the dark, painful feelings I had known were lurking. But there was nothing I could do, and so I just stayed where I was. Then, towards the end of the journey, the sun came out. It lit up the sky with a quite magical silver light – it was stunningly beautiful, and I felt that beauty inside me like a wonderful balm. But that couldn't have happened if I'd rushed off and filled myself with drink at the bar the minute I felt unhappy.'

Laurence does not think himself grandiose when he talks of that moment as a revelation. He believes it enabled him to see that he faced two choices at that time in life: either he could go on looking for sensations to anaesthetize the despair he was feeling, or he could find a way of sharing his feelings with others at the same stage and, through that, learn something new, while living with the despair as part of who he was then. Wilde McCormick believes that, if we allow it to happen, we will 'receive mid-life experiences' that are trying to force us to pay attention. Then, she says: 'We will be moved by the new experiences if we are able to glimpse their meaning and to incorporate them. If we resist any kind of change and throw all our energies into our conscious world, we risk becoming rigid, and the dragons of the past do not lie down but take the form of events or people around us.'

David Lyons talks of 'looking the demon in the eye' because he has constructed a concrete picture of himself almost as a mythical hero slaying a dragon. He explains: 'For a while I tried filling every minute of my time with social events. I worked ever longer hours. I flirted with women, hoping the ego boost when they responded would make me feel good. And I drained my family life of time and energy because that seemed the trap in my life. Briefly and spasmodically these things helped; they gave me a breathing space in which I felt a kind of renewal. But it never lasted, and then I was more despairing than ever. It was a friend who had been through something similar who helped me realize that I had to be brave enough just to acknowledge the fact that I did not feel a big, bold success, that I was floundering. I saw my feelings as demonic, and from that evolved a real, physical picture of a demon, like the schoolyard bully, who could reduce me to pulp by making me feel so rotten. I knew I couldn't run from this demon bully, so I had to look it boldly in the eye and say, "I won't be scared." '

Wendy Rhodes had her share of pain and loneliness after leaving an alcoholic husband as she was turning fifty, an act that was seen as folly and cruelty by many of the people she had relied upon as friends, so she found herself very much alone when she made the decision. In her words we hear what may come out of a period of grappling in the dark: 'This time is better than all the rest of my life because I feel I have been on a journey and learned such a lot about how to be me. I read the things I want to read now, go to the plays I want to see, visit the places that interest me and, above all, express the things I feel as my own views. I realize that during the marriage I bent myself and moulded myself to be a good wife and keep the peace, not to be too conspicuous or challenging. Once I got through the loneliness, I began to feel strong and free and very optimistic as, gradually, I began to do things I wanted and to realize there were no repercussions. Instead I could talk to friends about the things that interested me, and from that came conversations about deeper things and wonderful friendships have been born. It's strange to think I rather sneered at feminism and all the stuff about "supportive sisters" before, but now it's absolute lifeblood.'

Not everyone achieves such certainty or euphoria, but even Kate, the heroine of Doris Lessing's *Summer Before the Dark*, who tosses and turns in the bleak despair of not knowing from hour to hour whether she can bear to return to her family, eventually does so with a confidence about who she is, and how she will be, that was unimaginable before her crisis. The new optimism she feels displays itself in a dream: 'Her journey was over. She saw that the sun was in front of her, not behind, not far far behind, under the curve of the earth, which was where it had been for so long. She looked at it, a large, light, brilliant, buoyant, tumultuous sun that seemed to sing.'

Terry Neale too feels that reaching breaking-point enabled him to change. He explains: 'There was no way I could have persuaded myself it was reasonable to leave my job, even though I was aware of it being ever more stressful and less satisfying, if I had not become ill. When that happened I took a job as a house cleaner, which was wonderfully liberating. It was physically demanding and absolutely without stress emotionally, and it was during those days of Hoovering and sweeping that I began to feel a great sense of possibility, of courage. I took off for Europe, using my savings, and I travelled for some time. After that I went back to teaching and felt completely different about it. It was no longer my whole life.'

Leaving a long-term marriage that has become stifling and unsatisfactory can, in the throes of a passionate affair, seem the way forward, but, faced with making a decision, people often realize that this doesn't, after all, present the answer they were looking for. Instead they may opt for immense sadness, loss and grieving in the search for what Bonnie describes as 'a way to find my own authenticity'. She is the mother of two who pitched into black despair when, in her late forties, she fell in love and had an affair while still married. When it reached the point at which the affair must move forward or end, Bonnie looked at the pain she would inflict on her partner and children and realized that this was not what she wanted. She says: 'It was tempting, of course, because I knew I would lose my lover and that I would suffer a great deal of pain. But at the same time there was a curious clarity about it all: I simply knew that being with the other man would not deal with the discontent and loneliness I had been feeling before I met him. I realized I had to find some way to feel complete by myself, and to be stronger than I had been about doing things with my life which would be fulfilling but would not involve damaging other people.

'I think it sounds rather mature when I say it now, but I didn't feel the least bit mature at the time. It was intensely difficult after the break-up. I was in tears much of the time. I just wanted to be alone. I couldn't bear being alive. It was appalling pain – the kind of pain which, in the past I've always tried to alleviate. I didn't try to do that this time. I lived from day to day, managing – fortunately – to work. I made love to my husband by instructing myself to do so until, slowly, it became what I wanted to do again. I looked after the kids in a very functional way. And I read everything I could find that was to do with being strong in oneself. It was a very enclosed time. I literally felt I was existing in a time bubble.

'I remember during the worst time a friend said, "One day you will see a leaf falling off a tree and you'll be aware of its beauty. Then you will know you are getting better." It wasn't a leaf, in fact; it was a walk by the sea and being struck by how peaceful and wonderful it felt. From that day I felt gradually better, and now I can look back at what happened and see there was a point to it all. I'd never have achieved the sense of strength, of being able to make my life as I want it, by myself if necessary, if the crisis hadn't happened.'

Yet there are times when a marriage has run its course, and relationships counsellor Renate Olins recognizes this, although she warns that there can be intense loneliness and regret when we end a long relationship, particularly if it has been a family for children. But at the same time she acknowledges that in the case of a relationship where the heart really has died, where there is animosity, a lot of stress or a sense of being stifled on the part of one or both partners so it is not possible to grow or to feel any kind of contentment with a life together, it may be for the best to separate. She believes that couples who look after their children together, then decide to separate at mid-life, probably minimize the pain, and this is what happens quite frequently. And as we live longer, healthier lives and have a greater desire to live them fully and positively, it is increasingly being predicted that we will no longer regard marriage as for life but rather as one phase in a series of relationships or lifestyles. Ken Dychtwald, author with Joe Flower of *Agewave*, a thoroughly upbeat survey of the way in which, he believes, demographics will radically alter the way we live in older age, has cast this as a scenario:

We have the time and the resources to 'be' many different people during one extended lifetime. Some of us will continue to grow in tandem with our spouses throughout our lives, but many of us will grow apart. In the past, death nearly always intervened before a typical marriage had run out of steam, with decades of life remaining for each spouse. When people could expect to live only a few more months or years in an unsatisfying relationship, they would usually resign themselves to it. But the thought of twenty, thirty or even fifty more years in an unsatisfying relationship can cause decisive action at any age ... seen in this way divorce and remarriage are less an admission of failure than a shedding of a skin, a breaking of a chrysalis, a moving on to the next stage.

In Puritan societies – as so many in the West are – it is difficult to support the idea of marriages ending because people no longer feel they are good places to be. The till-death-us-do-part vow is held up to remind us what traitors to the cause we will be if we seek personal fulfilment – the modern Holy Grail – rather than old-fashioned self-discipline. There are, certainly, people who will ditch a marriage for twenty-four-hours-a-day transcendental happiness on a whim, and never mind how much suffering others must go through. Not only do I believe this to be a lousy way to live life; more significantly, I see that such people usually end up in deep unhappiness themselves. But that choice is very different from that of a couple who, having lived with a marriage that has been dead for some time, decide when their children have grown up to go their separate ways.

Richard Levenson, who left a marriage of twenty-five years, did so because of a growing sense of being 'absolutely suffocated, of my artistic heart dying. There seemed only two ways: I could either stay with my wife and keep the lid on my feelings or leave and cause damage and pain, and that is what I chose. I had tried for change within the marriage, but our value systems and goals were so different by this time, it was not possible. It was an immensely hard thing to do, and my sons, just emerging into adulthood, were devastated. One told me quite recently that he hated me and that hurt.'

For a man for whom family life was central to what he believes in, and who had been monogamous throughout a quarter century, it was a momentous decision. He wondered at the time if it were just a mid-life upheaval 'sending me slightly crazy'. Now, reflecting on the time since the break-up, during which he has suffered severe depression, guilt and has tried different therapies to learn about himself, Levenson talks with some degree of optimism: 'Things are improving with my sons and I hope, in time, they will understand that I did what I did so that I could like the person I am and feel some point in life. And I do have optimism again. The last three years since I left I have spent long hours at my sculpture. I have cut down my working hours and I feel alive, productive, in touch with something absolutely vital. I see my crisis time as having got me to this point.'

Mandy Walters has a relaxed, warm voice and the manner of someone who feels very much at home with herself. She is in her mid-fifties and has been divorced for nearly a decade. It was she who decided to finish a marriage that had lasted nearly twenty years. She and her husband Barry have two children, who were in their teens when Mandy began to feel 'a great fear of time ahead. I was living in this relationship where I felt the person I am was not recognized. I felt dulled down, that my strong character was unacceptable.' It was then that she said she wanted to separate. To outsiders it was a shocking decision: they had seemed a contented couple who had built up a pleasant lifestyle. Mandy says: 'I have always believed in communicating feelings, in discussing what is going on in a relationship, but Barry was very unwilling to do this. He wasn't communicative or demonstrative, and early on in the marriage I found that hard. But then the children came along, and when that happens your focus changes. I spent the years bringing them up being very busy, working as well as trying hard to give the children a lot of attention. It wasn't conscious but I think I made a decision about keeping my discontent on the back burner.'

As the children grew Mandy, increasingly, developed a life for herself outside the home through her teaching. Barry was away a good deal for work, and she recalls how hard they both found it when he was home. Mandy explains: 'There was even less communication because we didn't have the day-to-day minutiae. The children were becoming independent, and I realized that Barry resented my other life. He would assert control by being very domineering with me and the children when he was at home, in an increasingly desperate way – criticizing how I looked after the house or how I cooked. It was as though I had to be broken down. Now I can see how insecure he was feeling and how painful it must have been for him.'

The feeling that it was impossible to go on became over-whelming, but, Mandy says, she was also very aware that there was no happy way. 'I knew that separating after all that time, and with so much between us, would be very painful, and it wasn't as though Barry was a terrible brute of a man or as if I hated him. Nothing like that. Once I had decided to end the marriage, I knew I must prepare myself for a lot of pain. I was very clear that there was no way of ducking that.'

But even her decision to face the pain did not prepare her for the reality of what she now thinks of as 'going through a kind of bereavement which was much worse than I could have imagined'. They sold the house because Mandy wanted to change everything, and it was then, she admits, that she felt very scared by her own feelings of emptiness and unhappiness. She says: 'The worst thing was knowing that I was so needy myself that I wasn't able to mother the children in the way I knew they needed. I found it very hard to be alone in the house at night when they were away at university, so I went out a lot in the evenings in a restless way, but nothing made much sense.'

It was then that Mandy went to Sardinia and rented a small house, quite alone, for a month. She recalls being frightened at night by wild creatures baying outside, and she became acutely aware of how utterly alone she was. She remembers: 'That time didn't cure my unhappiness, but it did enable me to find the beginnings of peace, of knowing that I could be by myself and that I felt freer than in my relationship. When I returned to England, I realized that I could be on my own and enjoy it. Best of all, I felt a kind of flowering, the freedom of my own authenticity. I began to be aware of feeling happy and of expecting to enjoy life in a way that was very different from the constant anxiety that who I was would not do that I had in the marriage. And now I have a wonderful sense of peace and contentment. I have my home and my work and many very good friends. I learn new things all the time, and I see so many opportunities out there. I am also good friends with Barry, and he visits a lot. We have the children and grandchildren around when he is here, and although I know he would like us to be back together again, he has a better relationship with me now than when we were a couple.'

We can hear, through the voices in this chapter, how inexplicable the difficult feelings may be; it is not surprising that many of us feel the need for guidance. But we may not know how to begin to help ourselves or to find a way of understanding the process we have been pitched into. The importance of some kind of help in doing this is stressed by Dr Anthony Fry, consultant psychiatrist, who says: 'It is not just sympathy we need when going through a crisis, but some explanation which helps us to understand our own truth and to look at the central core dilemma we are facing. Only when we find this way are we able to move on constructively.'

So it is that people may turn, at mid-life, to counsellors or therapists, healers or religious leaders, to try to make some sense of what is going on and to discover a context for the shapeless mass of sensation inside them. Counselling and therapy – or, rather, therapies, for there are a great many different varieties around – are among the fastest growing methods of help to which people are turning. There is little in the way of concrete evidence to suggest how helpful these may be, but a great many people believe they have been helped, that the process has enabled them to get beyond a painful block. Brian Aldiss, just turned seventy, the writer of highly successful science fiction and erotic fiction, explained in an interview for the *Daily Telegraph* what he felt happened to him through the psychotherapeutic process as his mid-life decades were drawing to a close. Interviewer Max Davidson recounts: 'In a life of many watersheds, the most intriguing occurred when Aldiss was struck down by post-viral fatigue syndrome. His energy levels flagged and demoralization set in, to the extent that he would leave the house for his morning jog, wait until he was out of sight of his wife and then slow to a walk. Relief came in the form of psychotherapy, which not only cured him of his symptoms, but also enabled him to look at his life through fresh eyes.'

It needs saying, before we look further at what therapy or counselling may offer, that practitioners of these two disciplines come with very different personalities and approaches, and it is never worth sticking with someone who makes you feel bad (unless it is a limited and understood part of an agreed process you are going through) or who tries to control how you think. Over-directive therapists suit some people but make others very unhappy and leave them with a sense of powerlessness. In such cases it is right to exercise the prerogative of saying no and to look for somebody more satisfactory. Another reason why we need to be guarded is that anybody

can set themselves up as a therapist and advertise their services
– and who knows what kind of 'help' you might get this way?
Even if you have chosen someone with a verified training or
thorough recommendation, they may not be right for you. The
British Association for Counselling (BAC), talking about counsellors and psychotherapists, advises: 'You must trust your
own instincts and how you feel about them. Ask yourself if
you would feel comfortable telling this person intimate details
of your life. Do you feel safe with them? Do you like their
manner towards you and their attitude to your questions? Do
you trust them and feel able to be completely open with them?
The more open you can be, the more you will gain from the
counselling.'

There is a National Register of Psychotherapists of the
United Kingdom Council for Psychotherapy, and it is available
from the BAC. Even this register may not be completely fail-
safe, but it will at least provide details about the kind of
training practitioners have had, how long they have practised
and so on. There are many different types of therapy, from
approaches such as Gestalt, where a lot of emotion is brought
out, often in a very physical way, to birthing, which is supposed
to enable you to go back to your birth and re-experience
events that may have blocked your emotional flow in some
way. There is transactional therapy, where you make 'bargains'
with your therapist or with others in a group as to what you
will 'give' them and they you in return. There is behavioural
therapy, which is designed to help us change behaviour that
we recognize is damaging. There are analytic therapies that
take us back to early life, and many other kinds.

But getting to the point where we decide we will go for
therapeutic help may be as difficult as finding a counsellor or
therapist. We fear being seen as unstable, unable to cope or
weak, and, worst of all, we worry that we will be judged a
screwball.

Lesley knows this well: 'I have a friend who feels she was
very much helped by going to a therapist, and when I hit a

very black time in my late forties, she suggested I go too. I was drawn to the idea, but when I mentioned it to my partner he sneered loudly, and another friend said, as what was meant to be a joke, that she had always thought I needed a "shrink". But I persevered because I felt so wretched, and my friend recommended a woman whom I now thank for giving me some very valuable tools for dealing with life by myself.

'In the beginning I heard myself telling the story about myself that I wanted her to hear. It was thoroughly sanitized because, of course, I was wanting her to think me a good person. But within quite a short time I began to talk about ways I had behaved which I didn't feel good about, unpleasant feelings of jealousy, anger towards people, contempt – stuff I wouldn't have told anyone I knew better. That is the greatest thing with a therapist: you don't have a personal relationship. She would lead me on from the things I said, usually with a small, non-directive question but often one that startled me into thinking in a new way. It's a very difficult process to explain, but I felt, as it went on, that things inside me were unwinding, that the unbearable feelings were lifting, and I was able to feel good and more confident about myself and my relationships. And I found myself standing up for myself better in life. I felt much stronger as a person, and that feeling hasn't gone away although I gave up the therapy two years ago.'

Richard Levenson too goes regularly to a therapist in New York, where he lives, and sees the help he gets as the adult equivalent of being held as a baby. He says: 'I can go and shout and cry if I need to. I can be as bloody-minded or unpleasant as I want. Quite often I go in justifying myself because I feel guilty about the way I've behaved. My therapist can be pretty tough on me, but that's okay because I also feel he's *with* me, that he isn't going to disappear and leave me floundering. It is a sensation of being held safe, and that has enabled me to explore a lot of things that have happened in life, things I've done, and to work out why they went the way they did. The process has made me confident that I don't have to go on repeating the same things, and it means I feel more sure-footed now, in my fifties, than I have ever before.'

Lesley and Richard both went to psychotherapists to whom they talked and by whom they were guided into looking at past events and their patterns of behaviour based on them. I believe from my own experience, as well as from having heard it said repeatedly, that this process helps because it enables people to look at how they are dealing and interacting with the world. We may, if we can step back and look at the pattern of our actions and responses, see what impact they have and whether that is what we want. We can see how we may negotiate destructive and painful situations because of what we do, and then we can decide to change if that is what we want.

But how do practitioners working as therapists describe what is often seen as a process which is difficult, elusive even, when put into words. One practitioner, writing in America's *Modern Maturity* magazine, offers her interpretation:

Therapy is a way of speeding up and streamlining – or, even more important, unblocking – the process we all undergo naturally as we work to solve personal problems. It's the 'not seeing the forest for the trees' analogy. The psychotherapist acts as a completely objective overseer of an individual's problem situation. He or she is carefully trained to help the patient recognize and understand what's going wrong.

But where a doctor will feel obliged to try to make the client better, the therapist is not there to offer a 'cure'. Rather, he or she is there to help patients understand why they feel the way they do.

Liz Morrow, a manager at a medical practice now in her mid-fifties, had psychotherapy for eight years but stopped a few years ago. She thinks: 'It gives you a dialogue in the head which you can use to try to unravel things when they get blocked,' and, thinking similarly, Josh says: 'I see therapy as having given me tools for coping. It has taught me it's never somebody else's fault. Other people may upset you and anger you hugely, but you have a choice about whether you let yourself be upset. I value that bit of wisdom.'

Conventional wisdom has it that the young, with their flexible minds, their receptiveness, their relatively unformed personalities, are the ideal candidates for therapy, and that, conversely, change is something to which people are increasingly resistant as they get older. Myrna I. Lewis, a psychotherapist and assistant professor at the Mount Sinai School of Medicine in New York, has heard this often and disputes it vociferously. She believes attitudes are changing, so that 'We're finally beginning to acknowledge that people continue to grow and change at every stage of life. In fact, people in later life often have certain advantages over the young that contribute to the likelihood of a positive outcome in psychotherapy. Among those assets are life experience, breadth of knowledge, emotional maturity and interpersonal skills, to mention a few.' She is, she told *Modern Maturity* magazine, beginning to see more and more older patients, and 'I'm amazed at the quick progress most of them make.' British psychoanalyst Dinora Pines talks too of seeing an increasing number of people in later years and of the many ways she observes that psychological growth can continue throughout life.

But it does not work for everyone. Comedian John Sessions abandoned therapy: 'All those afternoons lying on sofas, wasting time when I should be President of the United States by now. It's nice, people with no answers giving *Daily Mail* analysis, and I wasted a lot of money on them. You have got to sort yourself out, and one side of maturity is accepting what you are and that there are some things you will not be able to change.'

We may look for help in confronting the dark corners of our lives, but we may, too, find that the best therapist is ourself. Writer D. M. Thomas, talking with Dina Glauberman in the magazine *i to i*, told how, after his wife had left and he found himself alone without family or children, he experienced 'a great writer's block'. He recalls: 'I didn't feel suicidal, but it was almost as if I didn't need to because I was already dead.' He tried therapy for a while, but gave it up and moved to Cornwall. 'She [the therapist] thought I was running away, but I felt I needed a new place – or an old place. I went back to my roots . . . Coming back has been a very painful process because some awful things have happened, some tragic family circumstances, but I had to keep going. I plunged into writing, which in a way was shutting it off, and then it came back with full force earlier this year.' Yet he has gone through that time, lived it on his own, experiencing the pain in a place which, with its memories of childhood, the roots intact, enabled him to remain quiet. Thomas talks of being more open now, more able to face himself as 'one of the great goods' that came out of his experience.

By the time we have reached mid-life we tend to feel childhood has been put to rest or at least has ceased to have the power over us that it did when we were younger. But unresolved childhood pains may be activated in a powerful, if not always explicit, way at this time when we are, in a sense, struggling to be reborn as mature adults. The profoundest infantile fears and an overwhelming sense of powerlessness which, it is believed, babies experience when they cannot control their environment and leads to depression even at this young age, may manifest themselves in mid-life. They may emerge as the intense anxiety and inarticulated anger we experience at not being able to control what nature is doing to us. Psychoanalyst Eliott Jacques sees us as being pitched into the kind of chaos and incomprehension a baby feels when he or she cannot get anyone to make the world all right, as our early adult defences against recognizing the 'inevitableness of eventual death' break down, and we are forced to face mortality. Understanding that this lies at the root of the pain and fear we are experiencing may make it easier to assimilate the genesis of the feelings, to accept them and, in so doing, take away their power to torment.

But if our childhood experiences were repression and suppression of the spirit, if we were not allowed to feel good about ourselves, or love was always conditional on our achieving what parents wanted or on our making them feel loved the right way, we may need to find a way to free ourselves of that legacy. It took actor Dudley Moore many years of 'being the funny guy as a comedian and kissing ass' before he acknowledged the 'grey childlike person inside who didn't feel all that funny at all'. It was in America that he turned to therapy for help, and he believes it has enabled him to put aside 'the bad stuff from my early life, the things that I see as having prevented me from having the confidence to get hold of life and say, "This is it." That may sound strange to people who simply see me as the successful comedian, but I believe that being a comedian is about trying to placate the world, and for years I died inside if I didn't get enough audience approval. Alongside it there was so often this greyness, no matter what happened, and as I got to mid-life it seemed intolerable. I've done therapy a long time – nearly twenty years – and I see it as a life support. I have no doubt it has helped me. It hasn't provided solutions – it doesn't do that – but it's tweaked at the quality of life.'

Elizabeth Wilde McCormick, who has explored the meaning of childhood experience with patients who have had nervous breakdowns, believes that throughout the adult years we can heal ourselves by undoing the pains of childhood. She talks of 'the opportunity to reclaim the child in us that may never have been fully appreciated before, never loved and encouraged, never allowed to have the whole range of human, childlike emotions'. It is an act of self-love which can bring great rewards, in McCormack's view. The way she explains it is that we may be able to move towards integration by trying to 'become' again the needy child in order to have a more satisfactory action replay. She says: 'This inner child can be held and given hope and life, and allowed to mature in the appropriate way that was previously impossible. We may then begin to reconnect with our natural path.'

Ben Rolands, who left a wife and four children, has spent many years since then coming to terms with the crisis of childhood which, he is now quite clear, cast long, dark shadows over his earlier years. He says: 'What went on in my mid-life was seeking to grow out of something else that had happened earlier and I'd got stuck with it.' He sits over frothy cappuccino in a north London café, a fit, trim man of fifty-seven who has jogged several miles to our meeting and whose enthusiasm for what is happening in his inner world these days seems boundless. He tells his story. 'The central thing is my being a twin. I was the elder of two twins, and my brother was undiagnosed. He arrived unexpectedly about half an hour after the midwife had left, and he was, as a result, brain-damaged. When he was six years old my father decided that it was not any longer possible to cope with him at home. He went to a private nursing home and, later, to a large mental institution, and he remained there until he died at the age of twenty-four.'

Ben was sent to boarding-school soon after his brother's departure and lived a life that took him further and further from any involvement with his brother. He trained to be a doctor and was busy working when his brother died. He says: 'I didn't go to his funeral. It was a blind spot, and at the time I don't think I dealt with the fact of his dying or being my twin.' It was afterwards that Ben began to see, through the therapy he was doing, how he had 'lived in the shadow of my twin and I did that until I laid him to rest which I did in a concrete fashion. I finally buried him. I went to the grave where his ashes had been scattered, and I put a stone down and wrote an inscription on it. I had a service – I made it up – and I said goodbye to him. And I was saying goodbye not only to him but to what I had taken on as constraints in my life because of him. For example, I think I studied medicine only as a way of assuaging the guilt that I felt about him and trying to make it right for my father.'

Ben also sees his marriage, which lasted fifteen years, as part of living with a script, a set of beliefs about what he should do, what sort of person he should be to please his father. But then, he says, 'It wasn't long before I had a sense of questing, going out and searching in a way which I felt unable to do within the relationship. I had a strong sense of being stuck, and the marriage couldn't survive that. It was after I left that I went into psychotherapy with a very dear man in Cambridge, and I started unravelling what had gone on. By now I was forty-three.'

It was during this process that Ben began, he says, 'to appreciate how emotionally tied I was to my twin still, despite my denial of it, and it gave me reason to understand my hostility to my father, my very deep anger towards him. I was very aware as a child that there was shame for my father, and shame for us all, in my brother being brain-damaged, and I don't think the feelings I had for my brother were allowed. There was no place for them.' He feels he had to legitimize these feelings through therapy, and so it was that he came to free himself from the past through the burial service.

Another way we may come to healing damage harboured since childhood is through resolution with parents, and it is perhaps not surprising that at mid-life, when parents may be close to death, an urgent sense can surface of the need to do this, to heal old wounds, to try to understand why love and approval were withheld. Critical feelings may well be triggered by the residue of pain or fury never dealt with, and the need to resolve these before it is too late becomes pressing. The incapacity to put emotional conflict with a parent to rest after their death is something many people who have not achieved resolution, or some kind of understanding, talk about. Sue, an office cleaner, had not seen her mother for twenty years when she died, and she remembers: 'I didn't feel grief, really, just a kind of realization that this was the end of an era. But then five years ago, when I turned fifty-one, I began to think about her a lot, and I started remembering bits of my childhood, and I remembered how unhappy I'd been a lot of the time, especially when Dad hit me about and Mum wouldn't stand up for me. I remember thinking she couldn't like me much if she wouldn't stop him making me cry. And she was always telling me I wasn't much good at things ... That was what I remembered. But then other things started coming up – good memories of when she took me on a holiday and we had a really good time; another occasion when she got me a bike even though I know she was very broke and probably, if I think about it, didn't eat for weeks to do it. It was weird: I felt close to her, and I so wanted to say, "Let's talk about those times, Mum. I want to know you did love me." I was in tears when that happened, and a few times afterwards. It still hurts, but in a way it feels better than not caring about my mother because somewhere underneath I did care.'

Robert Stephens, whose mother told him she had wanted to abort him and was, in his recollections, almost unremittingly cruel and cold towards him, feels that his failures in marriage, his endless doubting that he is good enough – in spite of his considerable acting successes – dates back to 'having all self-esteem bashed out of me as a kid', and he looks back on his mid-life 'bender' as a way of trying to blot out 'an immense pain that just seemed to fill me. I felt just the kind of impotence I had as a kid. My mother died some years back, and I haven't forgiven her – it would have been hypocritical. I think it has taken me until my sixties to push aside the legacy of my childhood and feel at peace with myself.' This happened when he met actress Patricia Quinn, with whom he now lives, and he says: 'She has made me feel lovable. I trust her affection; it is constant and nurturing. For the first time, since we got together, I have been able to get up in the morning feeling good about myself. So for me this older part of life, the prospect of going forward with Pat, is like a reward. I feel my mid-life crisis was like some dreadful, uncontrolled eruption which has now been dealt with.'

The pain of childhood for actress Lynn Redgrave was spelled out with dreadful poignancy when, at the age of fifty, she wrote and performed her play *Shakespeare for My Father* in an off-Broadway theatre. The play was, she says 'an attempt to look at and understand this man, who was not a hands-on father. He never ran to me and hugged me. I never really felt he saw me.' Indeed, the raw sense of this comes at the opening of the play, when Lynn, reading her father's diary for the day on which she was born, eagerly scans his description of the theatre production he was involved in, searching for his feelings about her birth. But there is nothing. 'Where was I?' she asks.

There were other assaults on her sense of self as a child. Performing in a school play once, the very young Lynn was delighted to see her father sitting in the front row of seats, and she continued happily. But, turning a few minutes later, she saw that he had left. When, as a teenager, she announced that she wanted to be an actress, Sir Michael let her know he thought she was without talent. It is noteworthy that, from young adulthood, Lynn battled with anorexia nervosa and bulimia, afflictions linked with low self-esteem, and as I listened to her talk, anger too dangerous to be expressed seemed very close to the surface. Yet when Sir Michael was dying, Lynn made a point of being with him, wanting in some way to be close to him before it was too late.

She says: 'The moments in hospital were lucky because I knew that I would never see him again. So it was as if time stood still. On the final day he became completely lucid and talked to me for the very first time about the rest of the family, and he put out his hand to me. That was momentous because he had never been one to make the first move. If I hugged him first, he would hug me back, but he wouldn't choose to do it.'

That was a watershed, enabling Lynn to get closer to the feelings she had had about her childhood. It was then that she began to look at Sir Michael's life, at who he was and why he was elusive, difficult, at times seemingly tormented, as well as an enormously talented man. Lynn says: 'I felt it quite difficult, when writing, to be close to him. On the one hand, you felt a kind of fury at what your experience of being a child was, all the things you said that were so unheard. But I was also able to draw this picture of him as a victim of what had happened to him too and to understand that he probably couldn't have been any different.

'The morning after I had performed *Shakespeare for My Father* for the first time I felt these huge sort of rods of steel roll off me. Not totally or for ever, but the emotional burden was light compared to what it had been. I didn't realize quite how much grief I was carrying until then.'

However difficult — and it can be very difficult indeed – we can help ourselves more than we realize if we reach out and strive for at least *rapprochement*, if not resolution, with our parents before they die. This is apparent in the words of actress Geraldine James, who, asked what her greatest regret was, replied: 'Not understanding my parents until it was too late.' Those who have done it understand only afterwards how much they were held in thrall by the pain of rage against the people who, they feel, should have provided the quality of love and care they needed and never got.

Jemma comes from a small town where keeping up appearances and not shaking the curtains of the psyche was what was done at any price, so she did not feel able to ask her mother why she seemed so disapproving and would not cuddle her. She says now: 'We talked about safe things: my school reports, what I would like for Christmas, what my favourite foods were, but never, never about feelings. As I grew into my teens I had a terrible relationship with my mother. We were at loggerheads a lot of the time. My father kind of faded out of the picture – he'd never been one for saying much, although I was fond of him – so when I could I left home and got a job in another town.

'Through my adult life we saw very little of each other, but when I took a counselling course I began to wonder what went on in her, what she felt about the satisfactions in her life, and I started visiting her and asking these questions. I thought she might throw me out of the house, but in fact she really told me things, and I heard about this woman who had been frightened of all her own feelings and desires (she didn't put it like that, but it was clear that was so). And I began to feel compassion and affection for her. We have become really rather close now. She's eighty-two, and I feel so very glad it's happened. I hadn't realized how much I minded not having a mum.'

Don says: 'It wasn't until I'd got free of a very demanding career and a tight family structure, and allowed myself to live among people exploring New Age ideas and the spirit, that I felt able to approach my father, who was a very rigid Presbyterian and who had been very strict with me when I was a boy. I went to see him just before he died at the age of ninety, and we had a wonderful reconciliation. For the first time in my life I felt really in tune with my father.'

It takes courage to be alone when we feel as though there is no centre to our being, and our strongest impulse is to surround ourselves with the singing, laughing, all-distracting crowd. Yet those who have taken themselves far from all that, gone through the fear and loneliness barrier and realized that being alone brings unforeseen calm and solace, often see it as a kind of salvation. Anne Morrow Lindbergh took herself off from her large family and spent time alone in a seaside cottage, collecting shells and meditating upon her mid-life stage. Her writings about this time, *A Shell from the Sea*, are a beautiful soliloquy on her changing state and, at one point, the business of being alone: 'We are all, in the last analysis, alone. And the basic state of solitude is not something we have any choice about. We *are* solitary. We may delude ourselves and act as though this were not so ... We seem so frightened today of being alone that we never let it happen. "No man is an island," said John Donne. I feel we are all islands – in a common sea.'

Support when going through a painful time often comes, for women, through friends. A tradition of sharing intimacies – whether it is the breathless speculation about a new male arrival in town of Jane Austen's heroines or the gritty stuff of Fay Weldon's characters in *Female Friends* – the experience of talking through feelings and problems has given women an emotional language which many find particularly valuable around mid-life.

Australian Patricia White turned to friends in Nelson Bay, where she lives, when her husband left her, 'a conventional housemouse', for another woman after twenty-five years of marriage. She says: 'I would never have been able to cope without the support of my women friends. We were a tight-knit group of single, divorced women who were always available and supportive. They helped me see that there was pleasure in being on my own, that there are good things ahead.'

Mira found the business of going through the menopause deeply upsetting, not because of the physical symptoms, which she dealt with, but because 'I hated the idea that I must become an old crone. That I must accept getting old, and welcome it, set up all sorts of conflict and misery. I didn't want to be that. If anything, I wanted high stilettos, black seamed stockings and lots of reassurance that I was still fun in bed.' Fearing it was a politically unsound way to be thinking, she kept quiet, dressed down and became extremely depressed until, she says: 'One day I broke down when I was having a drink with a friend. And when I told her she just roared with laughter, hugged me and told me how wonderful she thought I looked and how I was very definitely still a sensual, sexy woman. It was a wonderful feeling of relief and release. It allowed me to laugh at what had become a very private, rather dour fantasy. But then we talked more seriously about my feelings at that time, and I realized how thoroughly my self-esteem had been pushed under by the menopause. Somehow I'd bought the idea that one became dehumanized. After that evening I joined a women's menopause group, and that was terrific. There were masses of different thoughts, experiences, ideas exchanged, and I found it challenging, stimulating and very uplifting. Somehow we came to feel a rather special, very powerful group of women, and we spun some wonderful ideas for our future as reborn post-menopausal women. I don't think I ever did get the stilettos . . .'

The support of women was vital for Helen, whose crisis focused on the realization that she was not able to have children. She too drew support and comfort from the group of women she joined, who were in the same position, and she says: 'Talking and talking, knowing we understood each other, knowing we shared the pain, absolutely helped to get it out from inside me to somewhere else where it seemed a bit separate from my entire being. But what the group couldn't do was bring me to a state where I could see something else to do with my life. I had to do that on my own, and it took several years.'

The way she found was to breed the horses she has always kept and to become more involved with them. She says: 'Of course they are child substitutes, not the same thing but something wonderful just the same. There is an incredible bond between you and your horses, and I can now experience absolute happiness when I just go out there and ride.' She rides for two or three days at a time: 'I go for perhaps a hundred miles seeing nobody. It's just the horse and me, very much together, and we go through these canyons that are so steep and so rocky, then through deep rivers – sometimes we swim through them – and then across what seems an endless expanse of open country. The wonderful thing about this is that I imagine doing it for ever. The fact that I have turned fifty doesn't matter. I feel as though I plumbed terrible depths and came through, and now I'm very calm about things.'

Finding a way to talk through and share their pains is usually considerably harder for men, who tend not to open up their emotional sides to friends from an early age, as women do, nor have they had the permission and support to believe that their feelings matter that women have had during two and a half decades of feminism, a support system that Erica Jong, talking about her autobiographical book exploring her own mid-life, *Fear of Fifty*, spoke of as all-important to her.

So the intimate exchanges women enjoy are less likely to occur between men, who straitjacket themselves into a life even when it feels intolerable, when they experience the atrophying of all emotions or suddenly, apparently wilfully and irresponsibly, break free of everything without pausing to consider if this is the best way because the urge to escape unbearable, untenable feelings will no longer be held in check. This is something Victor Seidler, who has written on the work he has done with men's groups (*Men, Sex and Relationships*), recognizes well: 'Men have become so accustomed to shutting down that they have to really see the consequences of that to want to change. That is what the men in groups have done, and when we talk it is extraordinary what can happen – such a lot of emotion comes out and men seem amazed that it is all right to talk about what they feel instead of what they do. We need this as much as women and it makes me very angry that there is such a lot of sneering, usually by male journalists, who, I suppose, are terrified of their own feelings. But mid-life is a time when men need to be brave.'

There is a sense of something significant having happened, of a step taken in the right direction, when people dare to come face to face with their feelings and weather a mid-life critical time. And, interestingly, even those such as Michael, who related in the previous chapter how he left a marriage of twenty years for another woman and saw that this was not a solution, feel they have made a move in the direction of maturity that will enable them to take the next step more sure-footedly, with greater certainty about what they want and how to achieve it. The fact that one crisis has been dealt with does not mean other critical feelings will not emerge, but a point made over and over is that the experience of what one woman describes as 'knowing I could exist with my feelings, become familiar with them in an odd way, and come to experience a sense of strength and hopefulness' means they are unlikely to be so thoroughly subsumed in the pain again. And if we can make this vital developmental move, there are rewards that Professor Bernice Neugarten, drawing on her research into middle age, describes as 'a better grasp of the realities ... self-awareness, control of the environment, mastery, competence ... the conscious processing of new information in the light of what one has already learned'.

I have looked here at the demons that may torment us in mid-life and how we may find some way of coping with their impact, but this is just a part of what mid-life is about. I am not suggesting that it is a time of unmitigated pain and suffering. Indeed, there is much to suggest that mid-life is also a time of exciting growth, a new kind of confidence in oneself. Bernice Neugarten's research has shown this feisty, optimistic aspect of mid-life quite clearly. She talks of the Command Generation, as it has been tagged by *Time* magazine. The mid-life years can be a time in which the skills one has learned, the recognition of one's own worth, may be very rewarding. Neugarten's cheering finding from her research is that few people actually wish to be young again (although they do wish to *feel* young); that there is real appreciation of the ability to deal with life more effectively; and that 'Middle adulthood is the period of maximum capacity ... The middle-aged individual, having learned to cope with the many contingencies of childhood, adolescence and young adulthood, now has available to him a substantial repertoire of strategies for dealing with life.'

Yet it would be a mistake to see life as something which can be dealt with by formula. We may indeed overcome our mid-life critical times as they confront us and move forward, fortified by the experience, but that is not an end in itself. I sympathize with those writers who see gain and a new confidence coming out of our ability to go through the pain and struggle, but life will throw up other challenges and tasks, other, different ways of coping will be required in order that we may grow some more. Dinora Pines talks of watching clients growing emotionally and psychologically throughout their lives, and we should welcome this because it shows we are still alive in spirit, grappling with the complex business of living and therefore of developing. Jung spoke wisely on the subject: 'The serious problems of life, however, are never fully solved. If it should for once appear that they are, this is the sign that something has been lost.'

The point is that we should take on these serious problems and be brave enough to learn their lessons; we need to face the demons, find the best way of dealing with them in our own circumstances and allow ourselves to take pride in what we go through, knowing it is part of development and growth. We then earn the reward of looking forward with optimism to the next stage and perhaps getting closer to realizing what Winston Churchill believed, that 'The young sow wild oats, while the old grow sage.'

Will You Still Need Me?

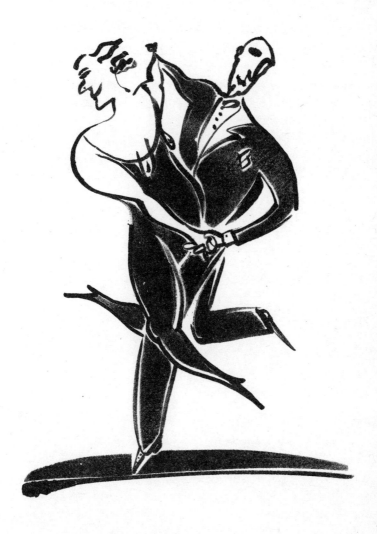

> . . . still I love thee without art,
> Ancient person of my heart.
> JOHN WILMOT, EARL OF ROCHESTER, '*A Song of a*
> *Young Lady to her Ancient Lover*'

WHEN THE BEATLES, MERE pipsqueaks at the time, gaily sang: 'Will you still need me, will you still feed me, when I'm sixty-four?' they could not have had an inkling of how close to the heart those questions are, as we reach mid-life. After all, as Freud and others have observed, from babyhood onwards sexuality is a powerful and compelling drive, an integral part of who and what we are. Of all the lurking fears this time brings, it is the idea that, as we age, we cease to be desirable, that the changes in our bodies as well as in our appearance, will cruelly and indiscriminately make us unlovable. We fear being and robbed of what is, at best, a vital source of expression and fulfilment enabling us to explore and experience intimacy, to give and receive pleasure.

There is plenty of evidence that neither desirability nor sexuality need end as we age, and Dr Michael Perring, a specialist in sexual health and director of the Optimal Health Clinic in London, points out that it is physically possible for people to go on having sex for as long as they wish to. But, as I shall go on to discuss, this is not how things may appear. My own received wisdom that, at mid-life the kind of sexual behaviour we assume during earlier life – meeting, mating, forming partnerships with sex as a key ingredient – is not what we can expect to happen, was confounded time and again as I was researching this book. Almost daily I seemed to be told some tale of mid-lifers falling in love, getting embroiled in chandelier-shaking sexual affairs, of older women with younger lovers and the other way around. Nor did it stop at mid-life; I heard many stories of septuagenarian or octogenarian couples who continued to have very satisfactory sex or who had begun new affairs and were outspoken about their good sex lives.

But while this may be reassuring in theory, it does not necessarily deal with the subjective feelings we have which are linked to our individual, private experience of growing older. Coursing against any amount of anecdotal evidence are, as we have seen in other contexts, the cultural messages telling us that sex is beautiful in the young and verging on the repellent in older people.

This perspective is particularly evident in the cinema where the big screen offers us a seductive and persuasive vision of life. As sexual mores have changed through this half century films have featured ever more explicit and transcendental sex, but always within a highly circumscribed field of vision.

Sex which smacks of paedophilia, or involves the most pubescent consenting 'adults' is big box office. The still taut, smooth-skinned thirty-somethings can thrash and howl on any screen you watch, *in flagrante*, but sex amongst the over-forties is on a fast-sliding scale and how often do you see unbridled lust among the over-fifties portrayed for public consumption? When we do, it is more often than not aberrant and dubious: the inappropriate lustings of a 'dirty old man', the pathetic cravings of a desperate older woman. The cinema has a virtual fade-out of sexuality and sensuality as we age. We may be led to understand, implicitly, that a couple of a certain age desire each other and have a sex life, but presumably detailed descriptions of thrashing limbs crumpled and rumpled by the passing of time, passionate kisses between those of pensionable age, are thought too unappealing to be graphically depicted.

How often does any of our popular art forms – books, articles, plays – suggest that older passion may equal young passion in quality at least, if not in quantity? Very rarely and, returning to film which has a particular impact, when sex involving elders is shown we are more likely to get some quirky tale of an ultimately pathetic Mrs Robinson captivated by a very young man, or the cliché of the older man lusting after a younger woman, than a character such as Susan Sarandon's raunchy, in-command older woman in *The White Palace*.

That said, it is interesting and encouraging, as demographic changes make it commercial sense for film-makers to embrace the desires and aspirations of mid-lifers, that there are signs of change. Significantly, in making the film of the astoundingly popular best-seller *The Bridges of Madison County*, there was much talk of how determinedly Clint Eastwood and Meryl Streep played the sensual and sexual scenes between middle-aged Robert and Francesca, with as much passion and eroticism as they would have done with younger characters. But more often, when we have the coupling of two mature characters, as in the film *Used People* with Shirley Maclaine and Marcello Mastroianni, both at the end of the mid-life era, we get bedroom scenes of such sanitized discretion that you cannot fail to assume the director reckons audiences will think this isn't really very nice.

The preoccupation from the 1960s onwards with all things young has replaced the old-style sex symbols created by the Hollywood studios. Jean Harlow, Marlene Dietrich, Jayne Mansfield, Victor Mature, Cary Grant, Douglas Fairbanks, may not have represented ordinary mortals reflecting the common man or woman, but at least they put across a powerful message of mature sexuality which was attractive because it was about life lived, experiences gained which could only add to what a lover would have to offer. Only the Latin countries in Europe present a more encouraging view with stars such as Jeanne Moreau, Sophia Loren, Catherine Deneuve, Jean Louis Trintignant, Jean Paul Belmondo, frequently given roles where their sexuality is considered as desirable as that of their younger counterparts.

I do not doubt that this virtual eclipse plays an important

part in affecting our individual feelings. What we see and do not see are significant in how we perceive ourselves and what behaviour we feel is legitimized. It is at mid-life that those working in the area of sexual medicine and therapy see how thoroughly confidence is sapped by the medium as message. Drs Philip Cauthery and Andrew and Penny Stanway, authors of *The Complete Book of Love and Sex*, acknowledge this: 'Many older people retain an interest in sex but fail to indulge it because they feel ashamed.'

Like many of my contemporaries, who pride ourselves on being immune to such obvious influences, I insist that my view of things is not so easily manipulated – only to find myself filled with a sense that I have failed in some way because I cannot go on being as sexually desirable as I was twenty years ago, that nothing I can do will alter that. My intellectual inner voice may tell me firmly that this is entirely natural, nor does it matter to me as much as it did, but nevertheless if I am honest I have the feeling that if I had done my personal best I could have done better in retaining a level of sensuality and sexual allure that is pretty much the Holy Grail in our sexually hyped cultures.

Yet my inner voice has a point. For, if we accept Darwin's theories on survival of the species – now enjoying a fashionable revival as they are re-interpreted by an emerging group of influential evolutionary psychologists – no matter what we do, we cannot be as sexually desirable as we go into mid-life as when we were younger. This does not mean older people cannot or do not attract each other for all sorts of reasons, and enjoy sex as much as their younger counterparts, but it does mean that they are very unlikely to experience the kind of sexual chemistry which makes people so irresistibly drawn to each other in early years. For in the scheme of things, where survival of the species is paramount, nature has designed a system which ensures that those of the ideal mating age, most likely to succeed in procreating and in producing viable offspring, are compelled and propelled to have sex with each other.

The male, explains evolutionary psychologist Robert Wright in his book, *The Moral Animal*, is driven by the desire to spread his genes far and wide in order to produce as many children as possible carrying his genetic imprint. The impulse for a woman is also to further the species, and she wants to make sure she does it with a male who offers the best chance of creating healthy offspring. These goals can best be achieved by coupling between men when they are at their most virile and fertile and women during their most fruitful childbearing years. So, according to psychologist Dr Julian Boon, who has spent many years studying the impulses behind human relationships: 'Nature patterns us to be sexually desirable to each other during the years when we are most likely to succeed in fulfilling her required goal which is procreation. It is all very functional and so no matter how well preserved or charming a middle-aged woman may be she is not patterned by nature to have the same pulling power as a younger woman. The same is true up to a point with men because they are likely to be at their most potent and sexually able when younger, but they can go on producing children for many years, and so in nature's design, they continue to have greater desirability than an older woman.' What we are experiencing is then part of nature's design but until we can understand and accept this we may feel as many do, a struggle to retain some part of what felt like life-enhancing sexual integrity.

Delia Watson, a forty-eight-year-old social worker, speaks for many women when she says: 'It is very important to me to feel that I am a sexual, sensual woman. I have been pretty monogamous within my two long relationships, but in a way I've used the fact that men have clearly fancied me, and wanted me, as a measure of my sexuality. Then about four years ago I started the menopause and I didn't like the way my body felt going through the changes, I felt very unsexy and it seemed to me that men weren't responding to me as I was used to any more. It was as though, almost overnight, something about me had died. I began to feel very colourless and undesirable even though I was living with my partner at the time and we still had sex. I realized how much I relied on being "told" I was sexual to be able to feel it myself.'

Peter Margolis, a fifty-three-year-old divorced solicitor, whose good looks and assured manner have made him extremely desirable throughout his life, found, just as he moved into his fifties, that younger women were treating him more like an amiable uncle than a potential lover, and women his own age who were interested in him, tended to talk more about shared interests than a shared bed. He says: 'I was at a dinner where there was a particularly lovely woman in her late thirties who I was very attracted to and I assumed she was to me, but when I asked her out she just smiled, in a sweet, not at all sexy way, and said she didn't think so really. That was my moment of reckoning. I suddenly felt I had lost it, lost my sexual appeal, and it was ghastly and deflating – I felt that nobody would ever want me again. It just seemed like an awful harbinger of sexual decline, and because it came at a time when I was worried about my potency the effect was very tough. In fact a rather older woman I met sometime later showed very clearly that she fancied me and we had a very nice sexual encounter which made me feel better, and I am beginning to recognize that the kind of sexual attraction of my youth may not be the only way I can feel myself a sexual being.'

It is particularly ironic when you consider that women reach their prime, in sexual terms, in their forties and both men and women who have had active sex lives through the years are likely to be more expert and skilful lovers in later life than in the earlier years. We are generations who have lived through the sexual revolution which, for all its imperfections, at least allowed most of us to experiment with sex and to have several sexual partners before settling with one. It allowed men and women to acknowledge sex as an important and exciting aspect of life. Why on earth, when our feelings and desires do not diminish, should we fear there is something not quite nice about our wish to continue being sexual beings?

There is no one simple answer. Cultural moulding of ideas, as already discussed, is one reason, but most obviously many of us are profoundly affected by the bodily changes which take place at mid-life and which signal to us, more clearly than anything, that we are ageing and that we cannot go back to being child-bearers or young studs with instant erections and enormous staying power. And, living in societies where there is no rite of passage for menopausal women or for men whose potency is diminishing, these bodily changes can be difficult to come to terms with.

Women at the menopause have, so often throughout history, been viewed as de-sexed in their bodies and unbalanced in their temperament and it is hardly surprising if we have internalized such ideas, often feeling as Barbara Martin, a statistician in her early fifties, felt, 'that nobody would want to make love with me because I would seem a dried up, crumpled up mockery of what is most desirable in a woman even though I know, when looking in the mirror that I have quite a good body and I still have powerful sexual feelings.'

And although men, as Dr Perring explains, do not usually experience the abrupt decline many women talk about during the menopause, changing hormone levels do affect their sexual potency making them realize, perhaps for the first time in many years, that they cannot be master over their own flesh. They may see the body they once perceived as their ally and source of pleasure as unreliable, taunting them with the shall-I-shan't-I dance of potency.

So the bodies we have displayed to each other, and derived pleasure from sharing in earlier years, too easily become a source of painful uncertainty at this time as changes begin to take place. What we need is to find a way to translate ourselves into the next stage of life, maintaining a sense of our own sexuality and sensuality in a different way from when we were younger. And before we go further it seems worth saying that plenty of people succeed in doing this and there is a good deal of evidence that many women feel renewed, more full of what the renowned anthropologist Margaret Mead described as 'postmenopausal zest' when they have completed the climacteric. It is harder to measure this in men because although, as I shall explore, the idea of a male 'menopause' is now being taken seriously rather than treated as a music-hall joke, it does not have a beginning and end as the change in women does.

Attitudes towards the menopause have certainly been altered in the past couple of decades largely because the women's movement has tackled the taboo on acknowledging it or talking about it, and instead has claimed the climacteric as an important and integral part of a woman's life and experience. Women have joined together to challenge the prejudices against menopausal women described by Germaine Greer in her extensive historical and contemporary study of the climacteric, *The Change*, as the 'sinister myths which continue to cling'. Women have also taken on the discrimination which, as Greer rightly says, still exists. We have set out to dispel the lurking idea that we become nature's neuters and shrivelled old harridans as our oestrogen recedes.

As feminists, who were the young pioneers of post-war feminism, have approached mid-life, they have set about reframing the climacteric, which is the transitional phase that may last as many as twenty years during which ovarian function and hormone production decline and finally end with the menopause, giving it a context, so that we may see ourselves as moving into a new stage of life. We may come to feel as writer Eva Figes has said she does, that the time after the menopause when she has felt full of energy and enthusiasm for life, is truly 'women's liberation'. And it must be some kind of measure of a change in public attitudes that Germaine Greer, in her menopausal years, has continued to be commissioned to write about her life and opinions, and has been asked to appear on television regularly, including fronting her own late night show *The Last Word*. In other words she continues to be seen as a woman of value. And equally significantly, whatever Greer herself might think of it, to be talked of by both sexes as a woman with sex appeal.

But while there are reasons why we mid-lifers may feel more optimistic than our predecessors had reason to about the way things can be for a menopausal and post-menopausal woman, it would be simply foolish to pretend that there may not be difficulties both physical and psychological.

Undoubtedly some of the ideas most likely to make us dread this stage have come from doctors who, up until a couple of decades ago, tended to be attributed a God-like role and any dictum uttered by them was accepted as unassailable truth. Take the deeply misogynistic – to say nothing of inaccurate – stuff peddled by Dr David Reuben who, in his best-selling 1950s book *Everything You Always Wanted to Know About Sex But Were Afraid to Ask* writes: 'As the oestrogen is shut off, a woman comes as close as she can to being a man. Increased facial hair, deepened voice, obesity and the decline of breasts and female genitalia . . . all contribute to a masculine appearance. Coarsened features, enlargement of the clitoris, and gradual baldness complete the picture. Not really a man but no longer a woman . . .' Havelock Ellis saw women at the onset of the change as caught in a last shudder of rampant sexual desire before their sexuality fades down like a dying fire, while Dr Robert A. Wilson, an American gynaecologist (albeit a quarter of a century ago), referred to the menopause as a 'staggering catastrophe'.

This is appalling stuff and manifestly nonsense but it has certainly played on women's deepest fears of what hideous transformation may be taking place. It seems clear that women who have achieved something in which they feel pride during their earlier years, whether that is being a parent, having a career, building valuable friendships, doing worthwhile volunteer work, educating themselves and so on, are able to stand back to some extent from the myths. On the one hand they have the confidence to trust their own observations that it simply isn't true, and on the other their identity is built around something more than their physical market value which, as we have seen, inevitably diminishes with age. Linda Ojeda, author of *Menopause Without Medicine*, is clear that research indicates that women who accept menopause as a natural condition of life and whose femininity has not been defined purely in terms of bodily functions – menstruation, pregnancy and motherhood – so that menopause represents the termination of their womanly identity are likely to find the climacteric relatively easy and to experience few symptoms. And they will deal better with the symptoms they do experience.

This is cheering in that we can look at our lives and attempt to alter the balance if we have become too invested in biological function and our roles formed around this, but we need to be cautious in being too gung-ho, for many women do not have access to the kind of interesting careers or opportunities to develop the stimulating lifestyles which may indeed boost their sense of themselves. The considerable research which indicates that women with professional interests, intellectual and creative outlets and challenging responsibilities have an easier time during menopause suggests a clear class and income division. That is made clear in the work of Professor Bernice Neugarten at the University of Chicago. In a survey of 100 forty-five- to fifty-five-year-old women she found that amongst 'enlightened' middle-class women there was little fear of the menopause: not many appeared to view the loss of reproductive abilities as too distressing and 22 per cent said they had not found the change anything like as traumatic as the myths suggested although there was for most some sense of disturbance. Most optimistically the women believed they would be healthier and happier afterwards – a finding backed up by post-menopausal women Professor Neugarten interviewed, one of whom declared that she felt like a teenager again.

But my research has certainly suggested that the reverse of this may also be true. Middle-class women deemed unenlightened or those who are not middle-class, may experience a drop in confidence and have a bad time with their change. It is clear that understanding and compassion for those women who find the menopause very hard is essential and requires resources to back the kind of initiatives we will look at further on.

It is also important that the menopause does not turn into a meritocracy – pats on the back for those who 'succeed' in going through it well, and pity for their failure to do so, for those who find themselves at the mercy of their physical and psychological symptoms.

We all experience the change in very different ways but more than 75 per cent of women are thought to have some symptoms which may last as long as five years, although these may be scarcely significant, sometimes no more than a minor discomfort. Linda Ojeda states that less than half of these women seek medical help. But there are those who find it very tough indeed and have severe symptoms such as hot flushes which occur as the oestrogen level drops and the hypothalamus sends out more and more hormonal signals in a desperate attempt to stimulate the ovaries into producing more oestrogen. There may be night sweats so intense that women wake up time after time in soaking sheets. There can be headaches which are hard to bear, insomnia, emotional unrest and depression.

Understandably we welcome the idea that it may be possible to banish these symptoms which is where Hormone Replacement Therapy, designed to replace the diminishing oestrogen in a woman's body, comes in. But how do we decide whether it is what we want, a drug which has been so powerfully promoted as the 'answer' to women's problems at the menopause, and indeed forever after, that it comes as no surprise to hear that it is the most prescribed drug in America, while in Britain and Europe it is used by an ever-growing number of women.

We have heard a great deal about the value and virtues of HRT and comparatively little about any downside, even though doctors in Britain, who are daily prescribing it more readily, were for some time pretty much split between those who saw it as the thing to give women at the first signs of perimenopause (the early stage of the climacteric leading up to full menopause), and those who adopted an entirely disapproving line and were reluctant if not obdurate about giving it, even to women who felt the severity of their symptoms made any help they could get worthwhile.

And there is no doubt that HRT *is* used by a good many women because they feel so much better taking it than when they leave nature to its own course – women who know that they may be taking a risk, and women who do not care for the idea of living on a chemical substance for years on end, but feel they have so much to cope with in their mid-life years that taking it for that period is worthwhile.

Clara Field, a nursing sister, describes a demanding job and fairly young, and even more demanding children, and says: 'I don't feel I could cope if I had to go through several years of waking up two or three times a night with hot sweats, feeling nauseous much of every day because of red-hot flushes, to say nothing of blinding headaches. These were the symptoms I had and HRT has done away with them. I don't want to take it for years and years but I want to hold my career together and I want to be a decent mother, and I don't want the fact that I've reached mid-life and the menopause to make things impossible.'

Mary Barton, aged fifty-three, and recently separated from a long-term partner says: 'It's been tough – not what I wanted – and then there was insomnia and hot flushes on top of everything. I got very depressed and I felt I couldn't cope with all that. After about six months of this I decided to take HRT and it helped a good deal, because as well as getting rid of the physical symptoms, it seemed to help the depression as well. I felt much more able to cope and see that there could be a decent future without Ben, whereas I'd felt absolutely drained out and exhausted before.'

One of the first and most enthusiastic doctors to treat

menopausal women with oestrogen was American gynaecologist Dr Robert Wilson who was convinced it could prevent the 'fast and painful ageing process' – a belief he saw vindicated when, in 1963, a fifty-two-year-old woman patient who had been following his treatment came to see him. Writing about her visit Wilson described in breathless terms: 'Her breasts were supple and firm, her carriage erect; she had good general muscle tone . . . her skin was smooth and pliant as a girl's.' Within three years, during which his use of hormone replacement was developed, he was declaring: 'For the first time in history women may share the promise of tomorrow as biological equals of men.'

With that sort of press it is hardly surprising that more and more women began to want this treatment which seemed to offer them well-being and prolonged youthfulness. And when it became known that HRT is valuable in preventing osteoporosis – it has been seen that up to 50 per cent of hip fractures may be avoided if HRT is started at the menopause – and that heart disease in women may be cut by half, many doctors began to feel its benefits outweighed the known risks. But there are other ways we can reduce the chances or severity of thinning bones and cardiovascular problems, and at a time when cancer is such a rampant disease, it is understandable that the idea of increasing risk, as HRT is said to do, even though the risks do not, on present evidence, appear great for women with no cancer history in their family, is something that worries us.

And HRT *has* had a troubled history. In the early days when oestrogen was taken on its own, a considerably increased incidence of uterine cancer was found. To counteract this, progesterone was added to the formula virtually eliminating this risk, but the therapy was then found to have brought about a small but increased incidence of breast cancer. A report in the *New England Journal of Medicine* (May 1995) produced new evidence of a link between breast cancer and hormone replacement therapy as well as suggesting that it heightens the risk of fatal ovarian cancer. An earlier study of 240,000 women sponsored by the American Cancer Society found that those who took oestrogen for at least six years had a 40 per cent increased risk of fatal ovarian cancer. For those taking it for eleven or more years the risk increased to 70 per cent.

This is all discomforting even though there are a good many thoughtful and careful doctors who say that, on balance, they believe the reduction of distressing symptoms, plus the substantially lower incidence of osteoporosis and heart disease outweigh the known risks. Others say they do not feel there is sufficient evidence for them to be sure just when and where the risk becomes significant and so we are on our own having to make the decision on the basis of what is known and hope no ghastly findings will suddenly emerge. It is hardly surprising that we may feel, as the first signs of menopause manifest themselves, that we are facing a game of Russian roulette with our bodies. As journalist Claudia Wallis, writing on oestrogen replacement in *Time* magazine says: 'Weighing the risks against the truly marvellous benefits of oestrogen may be the most difficult health decision a woman can make.' So it is encouraging to learn that a long-term well-designed study is now being set up by the National Institute of Health in the US. The study will involve 275,000 women, and they will be followed for at least eight years.

Not all women feel good on HRT and some actually experience worse symptoms than they naturally have. Some, like Marguerite Sander, a secretary in her late forties, feel bloated and put on weight. She says: 'I might not have minded the half stone I put on if I'd felt good, but I was like a basking hippopotamus – enormous, inactive and happy to attack anyone who came into view. It seemed ironic when friends were telling me they'd taken HRT to get rid of their irritability and how well it had worked. I stopped taking it after a year and put up with insomnia and headaches.'

My own experience of HRT was of getting PMT which

lasted longer and was worse than anything I had had throughout my menstrual cycle, and although I was glad to get rid of the hot flushes and waking in the night, the PMT coupled with the risk I felt I was running, did not seem sufficient reason to take a chemical drug I had some misgivings about. I was surprised, having made this decision, to find that I minded the flushes and waking in the night far less than I had before; I saw being able to deal with my body's behaviour naturally as a challenge. I began taking starflower oil, calcium, vitamins A and B and some trace minerals, and, whether it is psychosomatic or a physiological fact, I felt considerably better than I had on HRT.

A substantial number of women stop taking HRT which many doctors see as a prescription for life, after a relatively short time, while others go on and off it in an uncertain cycle. There is quite clearly a love–hate relationship at work, and Wallis rightly observes: 'For many women there is something fundamentally disturbing about turning a natural event like menopause into a disease that demands decades of medication.'

That was how Mo Harter, a forty-nine-year-old who is studying counselling and healing, felt when she gave up HRT and chose to go to an acupuncturist and also to a doctor specializing in diagnosing deficiencies in essential minerals which may need boosting. Three months into treatment she spoke enthusiastically about feeling a good deal better and optimistic that she could cope without HRT.

Increasingly women who have given up or who have no wish to start taking the drug, are looking for alternative ways to deal with their symptoms. Many, as I did, begin a regime of vitamins and supplements which are believed to counteract symptoms. And there are now many thorough and informative books which look in detail at a holistic approach to caring for our bodies during menopause – this includes diet, exercise and complementary treatments as well as vitamins and supplements. Natural health centres often have advice sessions or lectures on dealing with the change without the aid of drugs.

Getting to grips with our physical symptoms is clearly very important but, as already indicated, these are not the only thing which may make the change difficult. The psychological aspects of what is going on may be at least as important.

As I approached the change, I found myself reflecting with friends on our menstrual cycles, the part they had played in our lives, and trying to grasp that this all-important element in our existences, was coming to an end. We talked of the time when our periods started, the mixed sense of horror and wonder we had, the immensely powerful feeling of being a grown-up woman of having a place in the world. Vivid feelings came back to us, much heightened by the fact that what we were recalling, the experience of menstruation, was on the brink of becoming part of our history. And this preoccupation of ours was echoed in many of the interviews I have done which form the basis of what is said here.

Sandra Gerrison, in her mid-forties, unmarried and childless, finds herself reflecting on the choice she has made not to be a mother – a choice influenced by her own mother's parenting – and she is now aware that reaching the menopause and the fact that she will never have a child, may be more of an issue than she had ever considered. She says: 'I had a straightforward middle-class loving childhood, no child abuse, no skeletons in the cupboard. But I think that my mother was a good example of somebody who had not a clue how to parent. She was not neglectful, she was not cruel, she wasn't off dancing at parties. It was simply that she had no real knowledge of how to create intimacy with her children. Looking at some family albums, there's not one photograph in which my mother is touching me. She was detached and she stopped giving me the kind of attention which felt nurturing very early and I have always felt that as a parent I would replicate my mother's pattern and I don't want that. I do not feel I could be a good parent.

'I have had an odd relationship with my menstrual cycle, which is that when I was a teenager and well into my twenties it was a kind of absolute terror that it wouldn't come and the relief of seeing it. Now I still have heavy periods and every month I find myself thinking "Oh it's there again" and I am very aware of it, aware that, "yes I could still have a child", although realistically I'm not going to. When I stop and dwell on it it is quite an odd feeling that in about six years' time I'll reach the menopause and that will be that. It is an odd feeling and I imagine that what happens at the menopause is that you start going into some sort of crisis about your femininity, your identity as a woman, whether you have fulfilled it.'

Miranda Harding, a catering manageress in her late forties, voices what many of us have felt in different ways and with differing degrees of intensity: 'I had this absolutely stunning feeling of excitement when my first period came. It seemed extraordinary that now I could have babies, that I had a real place in the world. With my periods ending I have exactly the reverse feelings, that my place has been eroded, I am no longer what a woman is supposed to be.'

Jan Bernard is coming up for fifty and she expresses the perversity in her experience: 'I didn't like having periods at first, they seemed quite threatening and to put me at risk although I could never quite understand why. I suppose it had something to do with growing up in a very sexually repressed home where bodily functions, particularly linked to sex, were unmentionable. When I married and wanted children and had difficulty conceiving, my periods were a constant disappointment, so in an odd way there is some relief in the menopause, especially as I have had children. On the other hand it would be a lot easier if there were some kind of ritual encouraging us to acknowledge that the whole business of this cycle in our bodies has ended.'

Anna Watson, a counsellor who has been through the menopause herself, and has clients who do not identify their feelings of turmoil, loss of identity or sadness as having anything to do with the changes taking place, considers it important that we find a way of acknowledging that this time has great significance. She believes it helps some women to go through a ritualized process of mourning for the death of their fertility and adds: 'Realizing that the fertile time is past can be very hard although the reason is not necessarily that we wish to go on having children. Many of us, by the time the menopause occurs, have moved on from that phase, much as we may have loved it at the time. The change is involuntary, we do not have a say in whether we are ready for it and we may be trying hard to deny that it is happening. If we can talk with friends about our feelings, allow ourselves to weep if we want, to dwell on how important our fertility was, we may then feel able to move on and look at the constructive aspects of time ahead.'

Gilly Adams who began the menopause in her mid-forties puts it this way: 'I felt I was being thrown on to nature's junk heap. I would wake up in the mornings and rack my brain for ways to alter what was happening. As my periods got more and more infrequent I found myself trying to pretend it wasn't happening. For the first time in my life I longed to have periods. It is crazy really because I think I would be horrified if I got pregnant now and had to face the reality of fifteen more years locked into bringing up a child, but losing your fertility is not just about having babies, it's also about losing some essential part of oneself.'

For Maureen, an editor, her belief in her own 'youthfulness' has had much to do with continuing to be fertile. 'From time to time my partner and I have talked about having another child. I know it would be insane, I'm forty-six, but it's a fantasy around the idea that we are unchanging, we can go on being the same youthful people with the same place in the world, until we decide otherwise. My menopause made us both very aware that this is not so.'

It is not unusual for women like Maureen to feel inadequate because they lose their fertility and that, in turn, may lead to a degree of sadness or even depression which can then impact on our relationships and sex lives. In recent years women have formed menopause groups as a place to discuss such feelings and to look at and question why they should feel it is somehow their fault because nature has designed them to have a limited fertility span.

Suzanne expresses the doubt many women feel: 'My husband insists he is unworried by my menopause, but I find it difficult to believe that he can love me as much as he did. I feel that I must be less valuable than a fertile woman, even though I know Ed doesn't want more children. Deep down I know I'm scared he'll go off with a younger woman and nothing he says changes that.'

What we hear in these uncertain voices, and it can be heard time and time again, is women's feeling that they become less than they were and it is here that support and help for our psyches and spirits may be as valuable as medication. There are books which may be helpful but there can be particular comfort and help in meeting up with others experiencing the same thing. Lesley talks of how she has drawn much comfort from the self-help group she joined: 'I saw a notice in my hospital for a self-help menopause group which met once a month and because it was a friendly, rather informal notice, I felt able to go along. If it had looked like something intimidating and run by doctors I wouldn't have gone. There were about six of us and a sort of leader who just directed what was really like a conversation, so that we actually talked about our changes. It would have been so easy to chat about everything else. I found it really good to hear other women talking about the same symptoms as me, but even more than that I felt better when a couple of them said they didn't like making love with their husbands as much as before because they didn't feel very good with their bodies. That's how I was feeling, and I've put on a bit of weight as well, but the funny thing was, as we talked and laughed – there was a lot of laughing – it seemed much less serious and I've felt much closer to my husband since I started going.'

Grappling with sexual problems which arise from what is going on in the body is not, of course, what every woman minds about at this time. Indeed writers like agony aunt Irma Kurtz, a stunningly attractive, sensual woman, has written enthusiastically about the pleasure of passing the time of sexual desire. Jean does not have a partner and is unworried by the lack of sex in her life, but the menopause distresses her because it seems so clear a marker of time past and she says: 'It has made me assess what I've done with my life and compare myself with my peers and I feel I've missed and wasted too many opportunities. I know people say life begins at forty and look at all the things we can do in later years when we have more free time, but all I can see at the moment is a very definite end of what is, let's face it, usually thought of as the prime years, and I feel I'm just going to be a past-it old bird from now on.'

If we can come to terms with the way our life has panned out, then even if we find the symptoms both physical and psychological to be hard, we will probably succeed in processing what is happening and come to accept it. That may be less true for women who have very badly wanted children but have not been able to have them.

Judy felt her husband had only stayed with her because she had his children – she had had four, the last very soon before the menopause started. She says: 'When I began to miss periods I felt terror, an awful sinking sense of everything seeming to fall apart. The hot flushes were not in themselves so bad, but I felt my husband would see this as an awful manifestation of how I was drying up. I became very depressed, almost clinically, and I wasn't much good at being mother to the kids at that time. Looking back on it I suppose I was facing the insecurity I had always felt about whether I had any worth. Being a mother had given me that sense because my husband valued it so much.'

Psychologist Myra Hunter has done research into menopause and has run groups for mid-life women. Her aim has been to help those women who feel stuck with fear of what lies ahead through groups which question, and through challenging imbibed negative views, as well as those who are concerned by their physical symptoms. One of the things that came out most strongly was the sense that here was this new stage taking place but they didn't have the information or knowledge they wanted. It is the same in America according to the cover story *Time* magazine did on dealing with the menopause, and a 1990s Gallup poll of women aged forty-five to sixty found that only 44 per cent were satisfied with information they received from their doctors.

It was with this in mind that Hunter and her colleagues designed a project to measure how valuable informing women about the menopause and bringing them together to share experiences would be. One finding was that the impact of increasing publicity around the risk of osteoporosis and heart disease, and medical attitudes treating the menopause as akin to an illness, have led to GPs seeing an increasing number of women who are anxious about the change. Hunter questioned 178 women aged forty-five, and then divided them into those who took part in educational workshops, and those who did not but were studied as a control group. The aim in the groups, explains Hunter, was to 'improve knowledge, counter overly negative beliefs and facilitate informed choice about treatments'. She adds: 'We encouraged the women in the groups to look at their past and how they want to now balance their lives, how they can re-focus from their role as family carer and see the empty nest and no longer being a childbearer as offering them time for themselves.'

They also wanted to look at ways women might cut health risks by changing their eating and exercise habits as a way of taking charge of their health and lessening risks. Some cut down caffeine intake, the proportion of smokers decreased slightly. A measure of how successful this approach can be was that the participants in the workshops came out expressing fewer negative beliefs about the menopause. It was also significant that the number of women who had believed that experiencing depression is almost inevitable, changed their view. There was a decrease in the proportion of women who said they would use Hormone Replacement Therapy.

Hunter saw that, if women have an opportunity to learn about and discuss the menopause, to share experiences and to know what kind of help is available if the symptoms are bad, they are not just helped through the change but they are helped to develop 'life skills which enable them to feel in control of their menopause and which they can also use in later life'. Hunter talks enthusiastically of the strength and positivism which grew in groups where women, perhaps for the first time, felt able to talk about their perception of menopause, their fears, their symptoms, and to hear other women's stories.

The value of women supporting each other was also recognized by the Birmingham Settlement, a grassroots organization which formed a Women's Mid-life Experience Centre at the end of the 1980s, although when funding was stopped in the 1990s the groups ended. Women who came had hazy notions of what to expect from the change, and as they began experiencing the physical symptoms many felt 'isolated and robbed of self-confidence'.

An indication of how much information women wanted on the menopause was that out of the total amount of requests received by the Settlement, 50 per cent of telephone calls, 36 per cent of written requests, and 64 per cent of individual interviews requested were around aspects of it. They found a 'distressing' level of 'low self-esteem and low expectations from life during and after the menopause'. Many women, and especially older women, see themselves classed as 'second best' at this time.

Once they had identified the problems, the Settlement successfully used one-to-one work, group work and training to help women regain confidence and with understandable pride they note: 'We have had many successes – women moving into higher education, becoming more active in the community, doing volunteer work, setting up their own self-help groups, gaining paid employment, getting out of destructive relationships.' And above all: 'taking a pride in being mid-life women'.

The value of groups which can bring this about should not be underestimated, and one thing we should be doing is pressing for resourcing to have them set up in rural areas as well as towns where hospitals quite often run them. Catherine's story well illustrates how important education, discussion of the menopause and access to information can be, as well as support at a time when women are clearly finding things hard. She describes how 'it took several years before I realized that I was experiencing the menopause. For about two years I could not concentrate on anything. I was virtually unemployable, taking a job that was far below my ability. I was twice sacked for making mistakes due to my mental state. Being older, mistakes were not tolerated as they would have been in a younger woman.'

We may be able to help ourselves, suggests Gail Vines, author of *Raging Hormones*, if we stop looking at the menopause in negative terms, as a woman's lesser state, a condition in which we are 'hormone deficient' and see instead that the menopause has a practical and valuable role to play. Vines points to the work of Alan Rogers, an anthropologist at the University of Utah who, she says, 'portrays the menopause as an eminently sensible evolutionary strategy'. She explains:

Rogers' work is a sophisticated re-working of the 'grandmother hypothesis' whereby a woman accepts giving up her role as a mother and then concentrates on investing her time, energy and wisdom in her last born while at the same time building her position as a grandmother. If a woman continues bearing children into the stage when she is also a grandmother (which in any case happens fairly regularly), she significantly reduces the care she can offer to the next generation.

Looked at this way women can pat themselves on the back

for the important role nature has allotted as grandmothers. And the benefit of valuing ourselves in this new, matured role, is that it automatically makes the menopause a rite of passage.

This is not the only way the menopause can be seen as something constructive and forward-looking. Germaine Greer has spoken wisely, making the point that it is important we recognize that this time in life may feel momentous and that it is meaningful. The fashionable idea, often bandied about by women who do not want to be deemed slaves to their bodies – that if we don't let the menopause worry us it will scarcely be worth worrying about – could be just about as damaging to women as the bad propaganda. 'It is an important time and sufficiently so that in some cultures women are excused the duties in their community and allowed to go away for quiet contemplative times when they are experiencing the full impact of the change,' says Greer. How are we ever to get understanding and respect for what the menopause means if we attempt to prove ourselves so on top of everything that we wipe from the slate a stage which in many countries actually heralds an increase in status? Greer concludes: 'If it were true [it] would be lamentable, for the goal of life is not to feel nothing. The climacteric is a time of stock-taking, of spiritual as well as physical change, and it would be a pity to be unconscious of it.'

I agree with Greer, but I take the view about this as I do about so many of the issues we face at mid-life, where voices boom out at us telling us how we should feel or behave, that we must deal with menopause as best we can and in some cases that may mean attempting to feel nothing about it. Not everybody can or will frame it as a time of stock-taking – some of us may come to that later. But there are encouraging signs that women are going through the menopause and coming out bold, proud and determined not to be written off because they no longer have fertility to offer. Writer Sara Maitland has noted regretfully that there is no story-telling and mythology built around the menopause and perhaps that is what will begin to emerge. Meanwhile we might do well to hear more from women like pioneer Eva Figes, a contributor to Virago's uplifting anthology of writings around the menopause who tells: 'Suddenly at fifty I found myself enjoying a great sense of freedom, of serenity. It was the exact opposite of the panic and neurosis usually associated with the menopause. The change in me was striking and consistent.'

The menopause which so clearly delineates mid-life for women has always been viewed as both sign and symbol of our differentness from men. But in recent years that different-ness has become blurred as doctors talk of a male menopause, pointing out a number of symptoms they find in mid-life men who come into their surgeries which are remarkably similar to those experienced in women. Just as in women the oestrogen hormone diminishes, so scientists have discovered that the testosterone level drops considerably in men as they age. At the same time there is an increase in the production of the sex hormone which mops up testosterone so that there is less 'free' testosterone in the blood. This usually takes place during the late fifties to sixties and the symptoms men have often mirror those we think of as belonging to the female menopause: loss of libido and general lack of energy, fatigue, irritability and depressed moods, explains Dr Perring. There may also be stiffness and discomfort in muscles and joints, dry skin, sweat-ing and hot flushes particularly at night. In some men there may be swollen ankles and calf pain – all symptoms that women will recognize.

The difference, of course, is that men do not cease to be fertile, they are not faced with its psychological implications, but erectile failure and impotence can hit a man just as hard and humiliate him on top of it. Our sympathy may not be instantly at the ready, given what a hard time men have given menopausal women through history, but we may all benefit if men see themselves as sharing a mid-life process with us. And because they discuss feelings, bodily changes and particularly perceived failings, far less easily than women, the chances are they suffer alone and internally. Certainly writer Sally Vincent, in a *Guardian* article on the male menopause, believes so, talking with considerable empathy of the loneliness men may experience: 'The ageing process is as unspeakably vile for men as for women. Men sweat, they lose their beauty. They suffer the damnably humiliating side-effects of menopause. But men tend to keep their problems to themselves and to separate the functions of mind and body. When things go wrong they are inconsolable.'

It is only quite recently that these similarities have been identified, and some indication of how determinedly men may resist being identified with women's change is heard in the declaration of Dr Malcolm Carruthers, a consultant andrologist, who does not refer to the male menopause because it 'sounds wimpish'. He talks instead of the viropause. That said, he is quite convinced that it exists as a syndrome, according to medical writer Annabel Ferriman, who researched this new phenomenon for the *Independent on Sunday*. Dr Perring, who believes optimal sexual health can be achieved in a variety of ways, has researched the male menopause and takes the view that it does occur in some men and that some of these will benefit from a hormone replacement treatment. Dr Perring explains how over a five-year period 800 men aged between forty and eighty who described the typical symptoms were seen at the Hormonal Healthcare Centre in London. They described loss of libido as the worrying symptom, coupled with impaired sexual performance and no desire to initiate sex. There were also problems with erection. The men identified fatigue as ineffectiveness at work and less well-being at home than in the past. They also complained of sweating and hot flushes at night. There were some cases of accelerated ageing of the heart, stiffness and discomfort in muscles, dry skin, not feeling physically up to par.

Only the man and his partner will know how serious the bouts of impotence are but there are now various treatments on offer ranging from oral medications made from extracts from a West African tree, supposed to boost the flaccid erection to testosterone replacement treatment – the male version of HRT. And here we have the second parallel with women – that men are offered hormone replacement treatment. In their case it comes in the form of synthetic androgens and Dr Carruthers who has been treating men for eight years, believes, explains Ferriman, that this is a valuable treatment for menopausal symptoms. Dr Perring is more cautious and asserts just that 'in a proportion of the patients who had come to him', male HRT appears to be effective in restoring drive, sexual potency and well-being. This group of men, from their early forties to their seventies, in whom there are signs of premature ageing, 'may have a relative rather than an absolute deficiency of testosterone'. But Dr Perring, a man with a highly disciplined attitude to caring for his physique and health, does not believe HRT alone is the answer. Amongst the men he studied he noted that there was a high prevalence of stress either in the work-place or at home. In some cases the men were heavy drinkers and smokers, they had sedentary jobs and inadequate exercise. He is convinced that erratic eating and a bad diet all add to the male menopausal symptoms. He is a proselytizer for the view that we have a choice at mid-life about how badly we suffer symptoms of change and ageing and that dealing with the things that seem wrong may involve improving the way we treat our body, counselling and possibly relaxation techniques in addition. He says: 'Alongside the "window of opportunity" provided by a course of testosterone we strongly advocate lifestyle counselling.'

There are men who certainly believe they have benefited from testosterone therapy and John Smith, a fifty-four-year-old who spoke to Ferriman, described how everything seemed to be getting on top of him. He complained of a lack of sexual activity, irritability, sweating, and no energy or concentration and a fear of being out of work, as had already happened to him. He was given an implant and feels above all that it has enabled him to hold his own at work: 'I now feel I can handle things pretty well. I can still keep up with the young lads. I am working flat out [and] it improves the quality of my life.' Another patient of Dr Carruthers who was 'devastated' by not being able to get an erection is delighted by the treatment.

But there are certainly doctors who do not endorse the male HRT pointing out that there has been insignificant scientific research into it, while others are anxious that in men in their sixties who have small asymptomatic cancers of the prostate which if left to nature might grow so slowly that they would never be a threat to life, could have their growth accelerated by extra testosterone.

Fat levels in the blood can also be raised by testosterone and when we consider the number of men who are overweight and whose diets, as Dr Perring points out, are high in saturated fats, pushing up their cholesterol levels, it seems right that caution is usual. Certainly Dr H. B. Gibson talks of TRT, which is seen to restore a flagging sex drive rather than deal with clinical impotence as still being a controversial treatment which men would do well to take care when using.

Mid-life impotence takes a high percentage of men to their doctors and an extensive American population-based study, *The Massachusetts Male Ageing Study*, showed that complete erectile dysfunction increased from 5 to 15 per cent between the ages of forty and seventy years. It worries men a great deal, but it is hardly a new phenomenon. According to historian Lois Banner, Cicero in his treatise on old age, tells us that: 'Ageing men experience a diminution of the ability to achieve penile erection, a physiological reality known to early Europeans,' and a little later in 1948 Kinsey *et al.* charted a steady decline in frequency of sex activity throughout the life span of men.

But what is new is the recognition that men may suffer, psychologically, as deeply as women do over the ageing process and that sexual failure is the equivalent of their change of life. We should try to ensure, in today's climate which has become both more interested in and more sympathetic to men's emotional feelings, and where there is a greater willingness to see what men and women share in the human condition, that what they go through is taken seriously. Whether male menopause is an accurate title or not, the important thing is that bringing it into the open and giving it a label, legitimizes it as a male experience. Derek Bowskill and Anthea Linacre suggest that men's sense of becoming less of a person when their potency appears at risk is every bit as great as women's similar feelings at the menopause: 'The male menopause for some . . . is a terrible nightmare. What were once virtues and worthwhile attributes of middle age no longer stand as consolations for the fear or grief of a possibly waning virility.'

Little attention has been paid to this aspect of manhood unless the man runs off with a much younger woman in which case he is likely to get slammed by women of his own age and the nudge-nudge treatment from other men while, behind his back, the suggestion will be put about that this is the only way he can 'make it'. Not for them the support women tend to give each other when they act out their fears and seek what may be inappropriate fleshly reassurance – support which may help them to realize that they are not taking a route which will, ultimately, help them. Nor for men is there even the possibility of feeling pride in assessing the years of fertility and putting them away, which may be seen as the flipside of mourning lost fertility. Zelda West-Meads, a relationships counsellor says: 'Men's sexual fragility is an issue we should not ignore. Men have to prove sexual ability by doing it, that is so central for their ego, while women prove it by drawing people to them. Both sexes may be affected by self-doubt, but it cuts men to the core not being good enough.' And if we, as women feel the lack of ritual around the menopause, how much less there is for men whose mid-life passage is marked by failing potency.

Going out with a whimper rather than a bang seemed like the beginning of the end for fifty-six-year-old Bruce: 'I had always had a good and confident sex life and my wife would often call me a "great lover" – that did wonders for the ego and the other bits for a while! But I became aware of my sex drive seeming to drop a bit during the early fifties and then a couple of years on I tried to make love to my wife one night, and I couldn't get a proper erection. We laughed about it then, and I put it down to being tired. But when at Christmas we went on holiday and it happened three or four times, I couldn't laugh at all. I felt ashamed and such a failure even though Jane was sweet about it.'

When Graham Brown, in his early sixties, was unable to make love to the woman he had been seeing for some months he went into a spiral of fearful imaginings: 'I was convinced that I would stop being able to have sex. The more I thought about it the more terrified I became, and I'm sure after that my fear stopped me getting an erection. In fact I went to see a sex counsellor who just made me see it as something that happens and will happen, but not a permanent affliction. Somehow that made me feel normal, okay, and things improved. I'm aware that it has happened since and presumably will again but I don't feel so devastated.'

Just as women have recognized the gain there is for them in consciousness-raising, participating in groups, and facing head-on what the problems are, so men can help themselves the same way. Too often it is heads down in the ostrich position but they would do better to learn what normally takes place with ageing. This is the view of Dr Gibson who, in his book *The Emotional and Sexual Lives of Older People* gives a very lucid, medically detailed assessment of what the process of ageing means to our sexuality. He says: 'If men do not understand what normally takes place (a process that alters but does not abolish their sexual powers) then they fear that they are becoming "impotent" when they notice changes taking place.' This fear may well, as apparently happened with Graham, affect their emotional state so that they suffer from 'psychogenic' but not physical impotency. If men can understand that fluctuations and changes in their body will sometimes affect how they function sexually they may be less prone to what Masters and Johnson described as 'one of the great fallacies of our culture' where every man over fifty is arbitrarily defined by both public and professionals alike as sexually impaired.

The fact that sexual failure, contrasting with the early days when an erection all too often bloomed at the slightest provocation, tends to occur along with other signs of ageing, compounds the sense of having reached a plateau for many. It is at this time that they may, as Deidre Sanders, agony aunt for the *Sun* newspaper says, feel a deep regret and resentment at having missed out on the sexual revolution. They see what looks like adventurous and promiscuous sex on offer to younger men and then they look at their own thinning hair turning salt and pepper, the bags under the eyes, the too-large gut and feel anger at having been born too soon to experience what looks like the feast of uninhibited sex which later generations had. Then their son brings home a ravishing girlfriend and beats them at tennis, and the despair hits home with profound physical repercussions.

The man who understands that some degree of impotence is normal may be able to live with that and go on enjoying a sex life with the occasional hiccup, or he may learn to prolong love-making so that instant rock-hard erection is not essential. This is described as the plateau phase where the penis is not so elevated or firm as in the younger man. But Dr Gibson suggests the man who can make a virtue out of love-making in this condition may, ultimately, satisfy his partner more by not being troubled by 'the ejaculatory demand that may make the phase all too brief for some younger men'. A similar point is made by Dr Perring who has seen how men who can confide in partners and remain calm about difficulties, may then find that things change and improve. He says: 'I believe people can learn to change their expectations, to alter the way they make love where relaxation, gentle loving, savouring each other's bodies can replace an earlier style. Men then often find that they can last longer, that the quality of experience comes to light – I see it as bread upon the waters.'

Louise Mann, a glass worker, appreciates the change that has taken place: 'Billy and I have been together since our thirties and it's been a good relationship, but when he reached late forties, he became very depressed when he stopped being able to make love to me in the wild stud fashion which characterized our early years. It happened around the mid-forties and I really didn't mind because I love him a lot, and for me cuddles and enjoying each other's bodies matters a lot. But he couldn't bear it and went right off sex for a time. At first I asked him why, said we should try and all that, but it didn't work at all. So then I stopped doing that and just held him when we were in bed. One night we had quite a lot to drink and were all over each other in a silly, giggly way. He started to make love to me and I could feel he wasn't fully erect, but I made sure he knew that I felt very good with him inside me and he was very loving and in fact we had a completely new experience. Billy took a long time making love, I was very aroused and it was just as good, in a different way, from earlier times. The next night I told him this and it happened again, and in fact our love-making has moved into a very good new phase. These days if he can't get a proper erection he doesn't get into a state.'

For men who do not want TRT and who want help with their physical and emotional problems, sex therapy can help as Dennis, now in his early sixties, found: 'I failed to make love to my wife a few times, and the more she tried to comfort me, the worse I felt. Then one evening we had a row and she shouted at me that there might be something really wrong and I should go for help. That shook me and as it happened I'd read an article about sex therapy. I was a bit embarrassed but I asked my GP to help and he referred me to a big clinic at a London hospital. They were very caring and helpful and because they didn't see me as a freak in any way, and they could tell me how other men had been helped, I stayed with the treatment and things got a lot better.'

Apart from the benefits which Dennis talks about, a hospital

clinic will give any necessary physical tests, but equally importantly patients are helped to explore the time in life that they
are going through with all its implications. They may, too,
find it hard to accept that while they peak sexually in their late
teens and experience failing prowess in their forties, this is the
time women reach their sexual peak. That does not mean they
necessarily feel rampant or turn into the hottest little numbers
in town, but at some level men may fear that women their
own age will judge them harshly beneath the duvet.

The other change which may occur is a tilting of the power
balance. As children leave home women may feel lost, dependent and needy which can make a man feel valued and in
control, but it can also be too demanding in a way that turns
him off sex. Equally women at mid-life may feel a confidence
in themselves which has eluded them through the earlier years,
and this may be particularly true of those who have emerged
from the all-absorbing, all-consuming business of bringing up
children and very possibly working at the same time, so that
there is little time for any kind of self-development. As the
children leave home there may be pride in having completed
the mothering role, perhaps having achieved a certain seniority
in her work or at least having succeeded in juggling both. Or
there may simply be pride, as Mel Green, a secretary, feels 'in
having learnt a lot about how to look after myself, how to be
a good friend to other women, to know why I hold the views I
do'. At this time women quite often feel a surge of confidence
in themselves, an entitlement to feel good about who and what
they are, and with that they feel less dependent on, less
susceptible to, men.

It can feel very hard for a man who defines himself by
sexual ability, to feel a woman's burgeoning sense of confidence at a time when his sexual prowess is failing. Some
measure of the fact that this is increasingly being seen as a
problem deserving attention and understanding, is the number
of articles in the press addressing it. This includes women's
magazines where the line is that women should be understand-

ing about what is going on. In one, 'How to make love with the same man for the rest of his life', very clearly targeting the woman, the male's sexual progress through different ages and stages of life is charted in a quasi-confidential style so that the reader is drawn in to knowing what is going on, what to expect, how to help when all is not well and what to do when the man is feeling insecure and concerned: 'He may be depressed that it takes longer for him to become aroused and he may no longer be able to delay ejaculation and so reaches orgasm too quickly. He may also feel he must reassure his partner that he still loves her by being the same man he's been for the past ten or twenty years.' But author Dr Helen Singer Kaplan, director of the human sexuality programme at the New York Hospital Cornell Medical Center, warns: 'He's at the optimum age for a mid-life crisis, so may need handling with care!'

The need a man feels for reassurance at this time may not be within the gift of a woman who has lived with him for many years, who knows him well, to give. As we grapple with who and what we are, the person close to us, however eager to be supportive, may be *too* close. When a man feels too closely intertwined with a partner at a time when he is feeling very uncertain about himself, the feelings can be frightening. He may fear his dependence on a partner. Many psychoanalytical theories converge to explain how men at vulnerable times in their lives may re-experience the pain and trauma experienced when, as young boys, they had to make the psychic separation from their mothers. And there is increasing evidence that boys who have been forced to break close nurturing bonds with a mother in the interests of growing up, who have been made to fear being a Mummy's Boy, so that they reject their mothers while still having a need for care and nurture, or, most extremely, who have been sent away to boarding-school before they have satisfactorily separated emotionally from their mother, carry in them the knowledge of the anguished feelings of neediness and dependence which cannot be met. When in a relationship with a woman they feel dependence, it triggers, at a psychological level, the primal pain they suffered with their mothers. It is a theory around which psychotherapist Adam Jukes built his book *Why Men Hate Women*, in which he explores the profound anger, rage and rejection so many men seem, inexplicably, to display against the women they have apparently chosen to love.

It certainly helps to make sense of the familiar retreat from a known and trusted partner to a new lover, which is the way men like William choose during their critical times. He says: 'My wife really seemed to flower when the kids left home. She got a better job, she started dressing really smartly and generally seemed to feel good about herself. And what happened? I started finding I couldn't make love to her.

'It wasn't that I didn't get an erection but I just didn't want to touch her. It was odd when we did make love I felt real anger with her, a feeling that she was taunting me in some way, but I don't suppose she really was. So when I met a woman, not that much younger than me but very flirty and come on, very obviously fancying me, I felt terrific. The feeling was like a fix and I fell hard. We had an affair, a pretty torrid one, and I'm sure it's the fact it was a secret which gave it edge, and it made me feel very good indeed about myself as a sexual being.

'Then my wife found out and she was just so upset, she seemed to collapse – the woman I'd seen as feeling so good about herself was in bits because she thought she was losing me. I won't pretend it was like the movies and we fell into each other's arms and lived happily ever after. In fact it took months of re-building any kind of trust, but I realized very clearly that I wanted to be with Anna. And what did come out of all this was that I told her how I'd been feeling and she was amazed but I think it helped her to come closer to me, the fact that I'd felt she was so impressive and because I saw how much she did want me, I felt safer with her.'

For Lewis Barnett feelings which, he feels certain were a

desperate attempt to know he could be sure of his wife's love for him, a love he found it hard to believe in, led him into an affair. He explains: 'I had always needed more sex and physical demonstrativeness than my wife had been able to give, but from forty onwards this need became stronger. It did not at first result in the pursuit of an extra-marital affair – on the contrary, I seemed to become more and more desperate to get things right with her. But then the inevitable happened and an affair came my way. I grasped it as an opportunity not only to reassert my youth, my attractiveness to women and so on, but also and very largely, as a sort of megaphone through which to make points to my wife. There was a series of fascinating Freudian moments when my subconscious, although superficially I was trying to hide the affair, forced me to wave it in front of my wife.'

Sex is a powerful way in which people renew their sense of themselves and mid-life, when men's fears about their potency and women's about their sexual desirability may become acute, the need to do this may be stronger than in earlier years. Deidre Sanders is regularly asked for guidance by many people on this matter. She explains: 'I think it has a lot to do with panic in men as they are turning forty. Men who have been faithful for a long time suddenly start having affairs – often when I hear the details I see how it seems to link in with men feeling insecure at work and wanting reassurance and sex is the way they believe they can get it. Others, seeing all the stuff on TV, at the films, in magazines, all that wild inventive sex apparently going on around them, want the wife to wear a basque or stilettos, and when she's not too keen she seems suddenly very dull and they go into panic at the idea of all they have missed.'

The younger woman is a particular type of temptation for the man who, as author Gail Sheehy has found it sees 'nature narrowing his own sexual potential'. Therapist Kenne Zugman sees this 'attempt to buy honorary membership into a younger generation' over and over again.

He says, as Sanders does, that this has less to do with something being wrong with a long-term partner and much, much more to do with the man's sense of hopelessness and helplessness, his yearning to feel young again. Zugman says: 'A younger woman will seem, at least at first, the answer to that feeling. And we all know it: being desired by someone who appears to have what you want in life and who chooses you, is a great high. We are indeed re-charged, re-juvenated by it for a while. But of course a younger woman who is chosen as a way of offsetting the deepest fear, cannot possibly be the answer. She may be wonderful and a thoroughly good person, but the man has to tackle his problems, the reason his stage in life is so unbearable.'

But why a younger woman necessarily? One reason, Zugman suggests, is that it would be far harder for men who are feeling insecure about themselves to choose someone their own age. He believes this is partly because she will mirror back to him that he is no longer young, but also because a middle-aged woman is far less likely to take an idealized view of him, than an inexperienced young woman. Zugman has spent many, many hours listening to men who have found the courage to express their most anguished feelings. He says: 'I believe men acknowledge at a profound level the death of eternal youth and it sets off a longing for a closeness and intimacy they just can't have again; they feel the remembered separation anxiety and that I think goes back to two and three years old and manifests itself in the feeling: I need to be connected, held in the arms of a woman, to be accepted and cherished. These men are howling inside terrified that they are going to die old and alone. It's an infantile feeling so they go off and do what seems the thing that will help. They divorce their wife and marry the twenty-five-year-old aerobics teacher who allows them to act out sexually these yearnings and at a more superficial level makes them feel terrific because they can flaunt someone so obviously desirable as their trophy.'

Zugman and Jukes are saying that men, when they are

suddenly unfaithful at mid-life, when they abandon long-standing relationships because they have fallen madly in love, when
they set up home with a woman scarcely older than their
daughter, may well be acting out the most primitive quest for
what, in psychoanalytic literature is known as completeness.
This is the feeling of absolute closeness and security at the
most profound level which, it is believed, many of us last
experienced at the breast of our mothers. It is a feeling we may
spend our lives trying to re-experience, but it is at times when
we do not feel in control of the world, when doubts and
psychic pains disrupt our sense of security, that we may most
deeply crave this completeness. For men, a woman perceived
as offering the same unquestioning adoration, the willingness
to hold and to nurture without wanting an adult *quid pro quo*
relationship, may seem to be the solution.

Certainly Jonathan's analysis of his own situation seems to
tie in with this scenario: 'My mother went out to work and I
hardly saw her. It made me insecure and to some extent I'm
still insecure . . . you could say I sought security from someone
who adored me as perhaps only a younger woman could.'

But society does not spend time on compassion for the older
man who chooses the younger woman and it is easy to
understand why. In doing this they frequently abandon partners with whom they have established an adult life, so that
these women are left to deal with desperate feelings of rejection
and hurt when they too are at the fragile mid-life stage. Men
who do this frequently damage children who may feel shocked
and disgusted at the behaviour of a father they want to
admire, and very often they damage themselves. As Renate
Olins at the London Marriage Guidance Council points out, it
is a common scenario for a man who has left his wife for a
much younger woman to realize, once the overwhelming passion has subsided, that he misses the adult companionship, the
history they have shared, the deep knowledge they have of
each other. She says: 'What then happens is they ask to come
back and either the wife has been through the pain, moved on

emotionally and possibly has found a new partner too, and doesn't want to know, or they get back together but the damage has cut too deep, destroyed too much for it to be viable again. That said sometimes it works and the couple creates a stronger than ever bond because of the catalyst that has occurred.'

The married man who has chosen to abandon a long-term partner and perhaps children for a younger woman tends to be regarded as having behaved badly. But why should an older man who establishes a relationship with a younger woman, when nobody has been hurt in the process, be so despised? A measure of the kind of treatment this type of older man receives is spelt out in endless newspaper articles where the suggestion is that he is a repellent old reptile. Take this one from a thirty-something woman journalist contemplating the (now over) relationship between Michael Winner and Jenny Seagrove and what she sees as a spread of this unsavoury kind of coupling:

It is clearly a good time for randy dads to be casting off their cardigans and trying it on with younger women . . . we're talking fully paid-up members of old-codgersville like Richard Ingrams, Sir Terence Conran and Anthony Quinn . . . But it's the girls I worry about. They really let the side down. Why do they do it? I am thirty-two and the prospect of sleeping with anyone more than ten years older than me *max* makes my stomach turn. Call me narrow-minded, but my reservations aren't purely physical. Weird awful things happen to genitals. Awful ravages occur in the jowl department. Smells develop; tea smells, tweedy tobacco smells, denture smells . . . Don't get me wrong: I've got nothing against old men – indeed, I believe they can be very usefully employed as car-park attendants and as seasonal department store Santas.

For sheer ageist nastiness on any count this kind of stuff takes some beating, but it is also age-fascist, condemning every and any partnership where the man is considerably older than the woman, regardless of how they both may *feel* and even though they are consenting adults presumably making a choice. Why is this? Jonathan, who married a twenty-three-year-old seventeen years his junior, believes it is because of the power imbalance between men and women which automatically makes the older man into an overpowering seducer: 'Many people think that men who marry much younger women are immoral, that they have somehow abused their power and acted perversely.'

Yet not all marriages between older men and younger women are necessarily the archetypal search for ego massage, but may, like any other coming together, be one of those permutations of human chemistry and affection which lead us into all kinds of relationships. Most of us can probably point to at least a couple of examples where the marriage clearly fulfils what both want, where they have found a level of companionship that works for them, where sharing children brings a closeness that works. A good example was Arthur Miller with Inge Morath. In his autobiography *Timebends* he describes the closeness forged by respect for each other's work, and touchingly he talks of his enjoyment of what they share as parents – a revelation for Miller second time around. Publisher Anthony Blond, in his late sixties has been married to Laura Hesketh for fourteen years. She contemplates their situation: 'I do think it's a good thing, in many ways, to marry someone older than oneself. Anthony has taught me so much. He's urbane and original and such good company. People are too narrow-minded; they love to bitch and pick holes. I know they did that about us, because I was told about it afterwards. They said it wouldn't last.' And Blond fills in the details: 'It's not at all tiring for an older man to keep up with a younger wife. You mustn't imagine that a big age difference affects erotic behaviour.'

Annabel Moxon, who runs a bookshop and was coming up for thirty when she married a man of nearly fifty, does not think she was a 'trophy', but what she does think is that marriages with this kind of imbalance are about a 'trade-off'. She says, 'The men of my own age who I met seemed to be looking for someone to mother them and frankly I felt much more grown up than them. I couldn't have imagined settling with any I met. Douglas was at a dinner party and we sat next to each other and I thought him a very witty conversationalist and I was excited by his knowledge, his confidence about his ideas. I never had wild sexual feelings about him, not even when we decided to get married, but I felt very protected by him, very cared for, and it was quite clear that he felt charmed by my inexperience and he delighted in being a mentor. It really was a bargain – I got what I wanted and he the same, as he still tells me – that's fifteen years on. I do sometimes wonder what it would be like now to be with a man my own age, but I see friends having such problems and I think I'm probably luckier than any of them.'

Counsellor Jane Hawksley is in the business of understanding not condemning. She comments: 'There is nothing wrong with a man marrying a woman younger than he is. Couples with a large age gap get married for the same reasons as most other couples – mutual attraction. For the man there is perhaps the added pleasure that he managed to obtain a younger woman, while she may be seduced by the success and money of a mature man. In the short term – the first ten to fifteen years – these marriages can work very well. But it's when the men reach their late fifties that the real problems begin. Lack of energy becomes a major issue. Women peak – both emotionally and sexually – when they hit their forties and may then be vulnerable to sexual and social gratification outside the marriage. That desire may be reinforced by a need to go back and re-live missed youth.'

Jim McIntosh, now sixty, declares himself happily married to Jane who is twenty years his junior, but he recognizes a problem in the older-man-younger-woman situation which he had not contemplated when he first got together with the woman who had been a student of his and was, he says, in a very vulnerable state. He revelled in his role as tutor and comforter to her dependent student state. That was how it was when they got married. Now, ten years on, a fundamental change has taken place – Jane has grown up and McIntosh reflects on the change from when she turned to him for guidance and ideas to the time when 'she began to practise assertive skills, to become mature and independent. My career was over; hers was blossoming. Her life was a promise; mine was becoming a memory.'

In spite of this, he says, they have a strong bond and affection, and yet there is a sense that he harbours fear of what will come. And hearing the voice of a man recognizing that he is vulnerable, because he may suddenly seem an old man while his wife is still relatively young, is surely as poignant as those feelings expressed by anyone else? Do we assume that all men who choose younger women are charlatans who deserve their come-uppance? It is clearly not so. There are good reasons as we have seen why these couplings are often not such a good idea and will end in tears, and it seems important that men have this knowledge but that does not mean condemnation.

And what of the increasing number of women who have partnerships with much younger men? Hannah Brett, a solicitor with a partner twenty-five years her junior does not regard it as more problematic than other relationships, just different. She says: 'The age gap has been tricky at times . . . I felt very strange at first because I have sons and I felt uneasy, but Joe is remarkably mature and so very different to the sons and he was so determined that he wanted me, we got past that stage.

'I don't like the fact that I can't talk about eras past with him, because he hasn't lived it. There are those things, but far more importantly we have a very strong friendship based on the things we do together. I enjoy his vitality, and because I'm pretty vital myself I keep up! Sex is marvellous. Is it immoral? Am I cradle-snatching? I don't think so. Joe was the one who pursued me and made a choice.'

Amanda Smith is in her late forties. She does not analyse the reasons she and Jason, fourteen years younger, are together but says: 'We met, fancied each other, had a fling which kept going because we found we enjoyed being together. It just wasn't different to other times with men my own age. I was divorced ten years ago so I've been around a bit, as the saying goes, and the thing I am aware of in Jason is that he is much gentler, less touchy about whether I look up to him or admire his masculinity. He takes it for granted that we do housework together, that sort of thing. He doesn't get worried if I'm sexually dominant ... I like the fact he's from a different generation, and in turn I think he likes the fact that I have a fairly strong sense of who I am and have lived a bit. Call it a mother complex if you like, I call it yin and yang.'

Women do not come in for the kind of searing sexist attack and contempt meted out to their male counterparts, but there is certainly a tradition of criticism of this unorthodoxy. When Lois Banner, Professor of History at the University of California, 'chanced into a relationship with a man of thirty' when she was forty-eight, she was aware of society's disapproval and that set her thinking about how she had always considered cross-age relationships as 'a male prerogative unavailable to ageing women' and had been fiercely critical of them. She says: 'I had construed it as a quintessential example of sexism, a final ironic proof of the unequal access to privilege and power between men and women.' That was five years ago, and since that time Banner researched and wrote *In Full Flower – Ageing Women, Power and Sexuality*, a fascinating exploration of relationships between older women and younger men in fiction, myth, in history and the present. Banner asserts that things have changed so much in the past five years – a trend given public acceptability by the parade of showbusiness women proudly displaying their younger men – that these relationships are no longer seen as risible. And Banner sees in this a logical and egalitarian counterpart to the draw of the older man where wealth, power and status had allure. She says: 'No less compelling it might be said, is its allure when attached to women. There is the appeal of ageing women who have gained wisdom and self-awareness.'

This is an encouraging way of seeing us, as older women, when the chances are that we will construe our maturity as being over the hill rather than the pinnacle of desirability. In Los Angeles a singles service has been set up which aims to bring together 'sophisticated attractive women and younger successful men who empower each other' – no suggestion there of the dirty-old-dame approach. Mutual Admiration, as the service is called was claiming a membership of almost 4000 in 1994 and was set up by a former air stewardess and a columnist on the *Hollywood Reporter*, both in their early fifties. They claim it is a bid for liberation: 'Older men make you feel less than what you are. Younger men are raised by more liberated women, so you can be equal with them.'

One of the attractions older women may feel for younger men, believes Deidre Sanders, is: 'They feel quite threatened by young women who are often more mature than they are and may be very putting-down. Older women have often learned to be more aware of feelings, more kindly, and they know what they want but tend not to be demanding and critical in the way some young women at least can be. A young man will feel safe and in that situation he may well flower. I get a lot more letters than I used to from women who have got much younger lovers. Women in their thirties and forties with boys in their early twenties. I think it has to do with social changes, in that the men in those cultures have been macho, quite tough and the women haven't found the relationships sexually or emotionally rewarding. A young lover is gentler, they are able to have an equal relationship, maybe for the first time. The woman may be able to be the sexual initiator. These relation-ships do often hit problems and they very often don't last, but women quite often see them as worthwhile because they make them feel good about themselves, they can see themselves in a new light if they've been through an oppressive marriage and the effects may carry on after the affair.'

The likelihood is, with women maintaining youthfulness in attitude as well as appearance well beyond what was normal even fifty years ago, as they go on being successful in careers and with the expectation of a longer lifespan, there will be more older women with younger men partnerships. But writer Christine Aziz made the point correctly and poignantly in an article in the *Independent* newspaper, that women need to be aware that these relationships probably will not last for life, that they must be enjoyed and experienced for what they are but with the knowledge that few men will give up the opportunity to father children.

I have looked at the issues around cross-age relationships which may need facing if we mid-lifers, at an already vulnerable developmental stage, choose to make such partnerships. But for many of us the issue will be what kind of relationships can we expect with our peers as we get older. How justified is the fear that sex and passion will become at best an occasional pleasure, at worst a non-event as we age? There are those who have no wish for this to be part of the afternoon of life, who are indeed content that sex should end, but others of us share the feelings of the poet Montaigne who riled against the idea of celebrating the demise of sex: 'I hate this incidental repentance that age brings with it. That man who once said he was grateful to the years for having taken sensual delights away from him . . . I could never thank impotence for the kindness it does me.'

We may return here to Dr Gibson who points us optimistically to studies in recent years which show that older people are now much more sexually active than was previously believed, while Dr Joan Gomez quotes statistics which show far higher levels of sexual activity than the British National Lifestyle's survey, the largest since Masters and Johnson's did. She claims that 75 per cent of couples aged sixty to seventy have sex, on average, once a week or more and it may be adventurous – 50 per cent say they do it in more than one position and at different times of the day. Ken Dychtwald at Age Wave Inc has been gathering data on this, too, and points to a major US study of 800 people which showed that sex is enjoyed into the nineties. Television too has taken time off from its incessant paean to the glories of the young and their sexuality, to show programmes about sex in later life. 'Will You Still Love Me?', a BBC programme, was one of several upbeat and inspiring such programmes on which elders talk of the pleasure their sex lives bring, while anecdotal tales of older people falling in love and experiencing rewarding sex are ever more common.

There was, too, every sign that sex and love are very much a part of the lives of many of the mid-lifers who told their stories for this book. Mavis Hoyle, coming up for sixty, declared: 'I'm madly in love and who said sex stops as you get older?'

Majorie in her fifties talks of the new lover with whom she has recently begun an affair, with the excitement of a teenager in love, and makes no secret of how good their sex life is. For Bill, the woman he met after his wife left him has re-awakened passion and that, he says laughing as though it were not quite proper, 'we are both coming up for sixty'. Geoffrey, in his early fifties, has no interest in younger women but, as a very eligible bachelor, has a number of 'women friends of a certain age with whom I have delicious uncomplicated sex'.

This is cheering stuff as we look forward and should do much to lessen the sense of panic and fear of loss at mid-life which can make us suffer so much. The bodily changes which take place can also engender a sense of panic and lead us into unsatisfactory relationships in the quest to allay deep fears. It is time we looked into these issues and thought about their implications. Are we choosing partners of a different genera-tion as a reaction to menopause and sexual failure, in the hope that we can be renewed through someone far removed from our own age group? For while there may be love across the barriers, forged on the soundest basis, very often the quest for young flesh, and a younger stage of life, which seems to promise that we can, through osmosis, become the same, is in fact a manifestation of our alienation from our bodies at this time of change. Perhaps if, instead of going into spiralling denial and turning away from our contemporaries – often those who have been closest to us and who are also maturing – we could draw nearer, then we could learn to fear our ageing less and see that it is not a dreadful end, but a step towards what might turn out to be a thoroughly satisfying season of mellow fruitfulness.

Living Like I Do

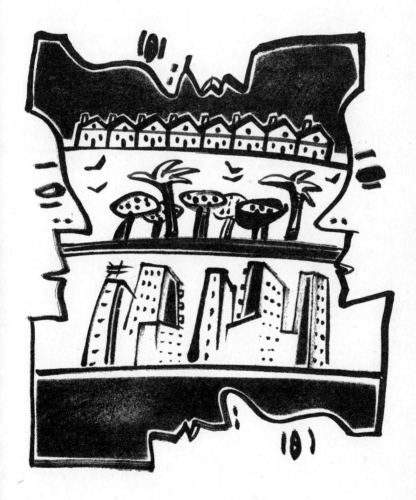

Home is where the heart is.
Proverb

THE CONVERSATION IS spirited, noisy, full of interjections and sudden howls of laughter. Some twenty of us are gathered around the table: men and women, from all different classes and backgrounds. We are contemplating the future, discussing a vision. The bond is friendship but the reason that we have come together at this time is that we have all reached mid-life and have begun to wonder about how we will be living in ten, twenty, thirty years' time. It is an informal discussion, what we all see as part of a process of exploring possibilities. We are talking around the idea of all living together in a big house, which we might buy through selling our existing homes. Would we have communal areas or total privacy and just physical closeness? Would we want to be involved in buying or renting homes in the same village or flats in the same block? Someone talks of lobbying a local housing association to let us help design a cluster of homes the way we want them. Someone else suggests buying land and building homes on it. There are plenty of ideas and, for all the lightheartedness, serious intent.

On another occasion I find myself airing the subject with other friends and these discussions throw up different ideas. Bob Johns, in his early fifties, likes the idea of a group of friends buying or renting places and moving into the same small town or village, while fashion designer Katharine Hamnett tosses in the idea of several good mates buying *haciendas* on the coast of Spain or a ramshackle house in the Italian hills.

She believes: 'There is a great yearning for a community and the intimacy this brings. People watch soaps on television because, subconsciously, they long for some place they belong, where they feel wanted and cared about, and where they have a role. That isn't just there for us so we have to create it and I believe in thinking beyond just staying where we are. Ageing in a warm country would be a much happier experience than doing it in freezing Britain, and a group of people who had bought the place to live in could exist very cheaply.'

I find myself sitting on a blanket in the garden of a young mother I scarcely know, in Totnes in Devon – a town where there is a strong culture of looking at alternatives to the conventional way of living – talking about how two people she knows, both in their forties, have just bought big houses with the intention of setting up households of like-minded people from the area and perhaps setting up courses based on the skills they have between them.

Later that day another person tells how her parents who had decided to sell their family home because it was becoming too expensive to run, and who had been daunted at the idea of having to re-establish themselves among strangers, have now found two other couples, people they have known some years, who want to do the same and they are looking at retirement homes in the same development.

Our ideas are, as yet, embryonic and we are not sure when we might feel ready to leave the more separate lives we now lead with their focus on individual families and work. But we all feel a time will come probably around the end of the mid-life period, when, with children presumably gone, and careers – at least those where we are employees – approaching retirement, when our foci will be very different.

The thing we all feel, vehemently, is that we do not want to be dependent on our children either to offer us homes or to feel they must be our support systems. But at the same time we also recognize that we do not live in neighbourhoods where we can turn to others for companionship and support, because we have grown up in fragmented post-war urban societies

where individualism and privacy have been the guiding principles. The perfectly pleasant, chatty relationships we have with
those in our home streets would not be likely to turn into
support systems as we get older.

Instead we have to look at re-inventing a community which
will work for our generations and it seems clear to me that,
rather than bemoaning what no longer exists we have to be
inventive and see how community or communitarianism can
be re-created in a way that is appropriate to our changed
world. It is here that I, and many others are seeing friends and
friendships as the basis for this. After all, good friends are the
people we will continue wanting to see, with whom I for one
look forward to spending more time once the demands of
children and a heavy work schedule ease a bit. The friends
with whom I have shared good and bad times, grappled with
issues, formed loving and caring bonds, through many years of
life seem the obvious people with whom to try to create a close
community in which we will be there for each other in the
future years. This way perhaps we can offset one of the most
daunting demons – the fear of being old and lonely.

The impetus to discussions like this, to the schemes being
drawn up, the experiments in communal living already happening, the moves by groups of people to small towns, the
creation of granny flats where elderly parents have privacy and
closeness and yet can be far more involved grandparents than
when they are miles away, are a response to the collapse of
community as generations before have known it.

Throughout the post-war years we have seen the dissemina-
tion of communities and families with the breakdown of close
family ties and the extended family. The high failure rate of
marriages often means families move and lose what may have
been vital, supportive links with those they have known
through bringing up children. The post-war lifestyle with its
ever-increasing individualism, competitiveness and freneticism
has divided people in a particular way. Privacy has become a
measure of people's conspicuous success. The wealthier we

become the further we tend to move from other people into larger houses, living there with the minimum number of people we can manage. The communality of letting rooms or sharing a house is the thing we slough off as soon as we can afford to, 'revelling' in having achieved this exalted isolated status.

On the other side the recession which has hit people up and down the social scale, and has led to the re-possession of many homes, has, too, done its bit to smash communities.

Neighbourhoods where people might once have lived all their lives and known and cared for each other, are now so often stop-overs for families coming and going as work takes them to different areas, or a change in income means they can or must move, and so we do not often now come across terraces and streets which have seen generations live and die within a network of well-known people and daily companionship.

The mother of my partner, Olly Hoeben, who is now eighty-nine, lives in just such an area in Holland and he believes it has been important in keeping her alive: 'She lives alone but there are people visiting all the time. She has sisters in the area, friends she has known throughout her life who are just around the corner. The local shopkeepers know her, my brother eats there most evenings, her grown-up grandchildren are near and if she needs help there are people living above her. She enjoys her life, there's always a bit of gossip, she's very interested in what goes on in her street, there's always a story to tell. I am certain if she didn't have this neighbourhood where she and her friends grew up and where her lifestyle is much as it has always been, she wouldn't have had the enthusiasm to go on.'

Such matters may seem remote, in the context of our own lives, as we first kick over the traces into mid-life, a time when we are likely to be agile and mobile, involved with work and family, able to socialize easily with friends and living in a style compatible with all this. But by the time we have made the journey through these mid-way decades our situation can be very different, and the way we were living then may no longer seem so comfortable or so comforting.

Along with many of my generation, I found the sentiments in the Bob Dylan song ('Like A Rolling Stone') – 'How does it feel/To be without a home/. . . Like a rolling stone?' – wonderfully freewheeling at a time when putting down roots was akin to bondage, and security was a word to be sneered at. But along with many of my contemporaries I now value just that security, the sense of a place I want to be, which means I feel *at home* where I live. The question now, is how to have autonomy and the separateness we enjoy but how, too, to create a home where as we age those things which we prize so highly when younger are mediated by being able to have a lifestyle which contains closeness, intimacy, supportiveness and which means that, if we spend more and more time at home, we feel happy doing so. It becomes increasingly important that home is where our heart is.

And mid-life is the time when many of us see at first hand the loneliness plenty of older people have suffered in the post-war years, as they have aged in circumstances where they are, effectively, on their own. Mark Thomas who is coming up for fifty and lives with his girlfriend and teenage son, expresses it: 'I watched my parents and their generation be utterly reliant on their partners, living increasingly isolated lives as they became less mobile, and then when one died the other was desolate and lost.

'It happened to my mother and she seemed to shrink into her loneliness. I think if her life with Dad had been more open, more full of other people, her distress would have been less. I feel it's essential to do things differently.'

Jane Murphy, now in her late forties, grew up in the suburbs and she too saw a society which 'insisted on maintaining privacy' so that, she recalls: 'When there was a divorce or a husband or wife died, although some neighbours made an effort to be friendly, there was no sense that people felt intimate enough with neighbours to go and talk about their sadness or ask for support. It seemed everybody did that dreadful thing of keeping themselves to themselves. I think of the way my friends and I are on call for each other when the going is tough and how vital that is to my feeling okay. Of course that's possible at my age even if we don't live close, because we are mobile, fit and energetic enough to drop everything and catch a tube across town or drive for an hour if necessary. But I can see that doing this when you are, say, seventy might be more difficult or even impossible, so the obvious answer is to make sure you live with real friends close by.'

Not everyone sees the need for future planning but for many people it is the idea of bleak loneliness, living isolated from friends and family, becoming too frail to venture out and rarely seeing anyone, so that home becomes a prison not a haven which, as much as anything, make the prospect of ageing fearsome.

These darkest fears are constantly reinforced by stories in the press or on television of the fourteen milk bottles on the door-step of a house where an old person has lain dead inside for days. Talk of granny-dumping and the unkindness to old people in institutions, although the numbers in this situation are, in fact, extremely low, reinforce the fears, and no matter how small the numbers it is important that we are aware enough to try to make sure it never happens. But for us the question is how do we prevent those darkest imaginings, or even, on a less dramatic scale, a sense of being without purpose, where time seems hard to fill, from becoming reality? We need to see the possibilities for being pro-active rather than waiting and hoping that fate will be benign in its workings.

We must look at what is feasible, what our needs are likely to be and how they might be met, how we may have some say in what councils do for those of us dependent on state housing. We need to consider how our circumstances will change – children leaving home, retirement, a change in income, but also the greater amount of freedom we will have.

There is the very real possibility that many of us through divorce or the death of a partner will end up living alone. This applies particularly to women who are statistically less likely than men to re-marry after a mid-life marriage break-up and likely to live longer than their male partners. It may not be cheerful to contemplate all this, but in fact people who have done so and drawn up contingency plans often feel they have fared better than if they had refused to think about how things would be in changed circumstances and then suffered because things were not as they had hoped.

Anna Lewis, in her forties, is clear on the need to do rather than wait and see: 'The present generation of old people had the idea that somehow they would be looked after, valued in older age and that the state would consider their best interests, so they did not see the need to plan strategies as I believe we must.

'But the benign state turned out to be nothing of the sort and far too many old people now live in lousy housing, away from people they know and they are broken down by loneliness and poverty. I think it is important to get involved with local politics, housing associations, and become involved with the decisions being made about homes for older people. There are some good schemes around but too many bad ones as well, so it's up to us to make sure the good ones become the prototypes. It just isn't any good assuming things will work out for us, they won't unless we do it ourselves.'

Mid-life is the time when we may be in a stronger position than at any other to plan and prepare a living style for the future. We are likely to have greater disposable income than in the earlier years, particularly if the cost of looking after children has gone, or if we have managed to save a bit. It may be that a home which was right for a family with children feels too large and too empty when we are alone with just a partner or on our own. Looked at one way it is a wonderful opportunity to make changes and experiment with ways of living. Katherine Whitehorn, a columnist in the *Observer*, floated the idea some years ago of creating our own communities in an article called 'Growing Old in Groups'. The idea caught the imagination of Margot Kuht who went on to visualize in detail her own thoughts on how friends might create a 'community' with their own self-contained accommodation so they had privacy and autonomy but also closeness. She wrote this up and was one of a significant number of people who responded to the *Observer* article. She recalls: 'Meetings followed where several of us who had expressed interest in pursuing the idea got together, but numbers dwindled and in the end nothing came of it.'

Bringing such schemes to fruition may not be easy – timing, finance, and a genuine commitment are obviously the things that must follow the conjuring up of visions. Writer Claire Tomalin, in her mid-fifties, began to consider the idea of a place among friends but which also allowed for privacy. She and a dozen like-minded people talked of finding a big place and dividing it into separate units but keeping one or two communal rooms. There would be shared grounds with, perhaps, small private gardens within them. Writing about this in the *Independent on Sunday* newspaper she said enthusiastically: 'Twelve of us would be able to afford luxuries none of us could ever contemplate singly: a swimming pool for instance.'

There was also talk of a flat for a resident nurse, something many of us have discussed when contemplating such schemes in the knowledge they were planning for the years when realistically we might well need such a facility. The scheme had not happened at the time Tomalin wrote about it and she, like many of us, clearly did not feel the right time had come.

Tomalin, as friends of mine have done, began with the notion of a country idyll but then started wondering whether she wanted so radical a move. Instead she considered, for instance, moving into a mansion block in town.

Alys Kihl, fifty, is a friend who has thought a good deal about this and says: 'I already know three people with flats in the same mansion block and I have put the word out that I would like to know when a flat goes on the market. The idea of getting a flat there with my partner among the friends I already know living there appeals to me. I mind a lot about privacy and autonomy and I think a flat that was designed to be separate but where I would be close enough to pop in and see friends for a chat when I felt like it, and where there would be a sense of community is just right.'

Such dreams are seen to be the prerogative of the moneyed classes, house-owners who are in a position to raise the cash to pursue their dreams. But it need not be so limited if imaginative schemes such as that being drawn up by a group of people in their forties, in Northumberland, are explored. Jed Wilson, one of the initiators explains: 'There's a group of us, whose kids have all left home and we want to live together in a big place. Some of us have money, others don't. So we've drawn up a plan where those who are earning and have money buy a big place cheaply, in need of total renovation. Those who are unemployed but have time will do the work on the house and that is costed as their contribution. That way they will be part owners.'

Getting such schemes right, making them work and sacrificing the notion of individual homes which have been the goal many of us have strived to achieve in earlier years, will take psychological as well as practical planning.

But it seems clear to me that these schemes, if they can be evolved so that problems, rifts, ideological disagreements – the tripwires which are so often encountered – are minimized and can be sorted out if they do occur, are a progressive bit of thinking. Tried and tested friendships, the kind which have weathered storms and where the friends care for each other enough to want to get through the times when communality may throw up difficulties, seem the best bet to me.

Tomalin in her discussion touched on the virtues of living among friends: 'Growing old, we become more and more like ourselves, each set in our own view of how things should be, resistant to other views and people – group living might prevent us from ossifying completely. The friendships of old age can be calm and tolerant. It is good to mourn losses together.'

The human warmth and empathy are certainly an important aspect of such ideas, but there is another. The dynamics of a group can often achieve much more whether in physical creation of the environment or spiritual development, than can be done by individuals each working out their own way and perhaps losing heart because they feel isolated, out on a limb. This was said to me with zealous conviction many, many times when I visited the Findhorn Foundation, perhaps the best-known and best-established community in Britain.

The very idea of joining a large-scale community with the sort of strong spiritual ethos that Findhorn embraces is anathema to many people, but I was interested to see and hear from the inside what it is that draws people in and keeps them there. There are a good number of long-established members of Findhorn and, with the average age now in the forties, a pressing question is what they have to offer people as they get older.

After all, we tend to think of communes as a hangover from the 1960s, an idea designed to challenge the nuclear family and establishment culture, started by the young and fading into oblivion as they moved into more bourgeois lifestyles. But Findhorn which was, indeed, founded on an ideological high in the 1960s, is a survivor. Peter and Eileen Caddy talked of finding the divine in everyday situations and, with what plenty of people regarded as blind optimism, but what they saw as a spiritual challenge, they bought a plot of land on some wind-blown terrain in the north of Scotland. Here they battled with seemingly impossible conditions and succeeded in growing vegetables. They constructed their own home and started attracting followers keen to get in on their earthy spiritual development. People came from Europe, America, the Antipodes as well as from around Britain, to join the Caddys.

Over two decades the Foundation has become an established

centre for New Age activities, offering a kind of spiritual holiday-camp experience, where visitors come for brief courses but are kept in touch with the world of creature comforts: the accommodation is comfortable, the organic food delicious and plentiful. And this erstwhile Spartan experiment has become enough of a tourist attraction these days to have a large caravan park and holiday lets.

It is signposted well before you reach the community's own houses, gardens and grottos. There are shops selling handicrafts and a vast range of metaphysical and spiritual books, as well as the kinds of novels you might well find in railway stations.

But the enduring heart of the Findhorn community is its group of more than a hundred people who have settled there making it their home, living in houses they have built or which have been built by the community – the most enticing are round, constructed from enormous whisky vats. They earn a subsistence income by working on everything from building and physical work in the grounds to administration and running the huge range of workshops and courses ranging from esoteric-sounding New Age matters to the most temporal and academic explorations of ecology, environmental issues and philosophical studies.

The first thing which hits you is the *esprit de corps* of those who have made the Findhorn community their home. They tell similar tales of disillusion with the ways they were living in the 'outside world', the pleasure they take in being amongst like-minded people and there is much talk of the community being 'there for you' when you need it. The next thing that hits you is how sociable it is: food is served in a large dining room, although eating communally is optional, and people seem to have a remarkable amount to say to each other as they sit around the stripped wood tables, when they meet in the café, or stop on the highways and by-ways of what is now a spacious campus. There is a great deal of eye contact, hugging and feel-good body touching.

It is easy to pass sardonic comment on all this, but the fact is there appeared to be a great deal of enthusiasm for the lifestyle – although by the end of my visit I felt an urge to see what would happen if I became thoroughly sulky.

Lois, a divorcee who came to Findhorn 'in a bloody dismal state', her marriage having ended, children gone and, she says, a very painful feeling of emptiness in life. That's not how it is now: 'You feel so loved here, people really do care about each other – everyone does. When I came people made sure they spent time with me, helped me fit in, made me feel this was home, and I can't believe how happy I am these days,' she tells me with enormous emphasis.

Many of the people had, it seemed, come to Findhorn because their personal lives had split apart or because they were lonely, and most were clear that living this way gave them a sense of belonging, of being part of a lifestyle where they mattered and there was much talk of a sense of growing and of feeling cared about.

Terry, in his late forties, joined the Findhorn Foundation after 'a sort of breakdown' which made him leave a prestigious teaching job and his native Australia. He explains: 'Living the way I was brought up to believe is the right way – marriage, the nuclear family, a good job and a pension, barbecues with the neighbours at the weekends, and never getting too close, never behaving in an odd way – just blew apart for me. When that happened I felt desperate and alone.

'My marriage had broken up, my wife and I just grew further and further apart. In my search for some kind of meaning I had begun to read books with a spiritual line. I came across a book on Findhorn and as I read about this community with its sense of purpose, its belief that we can lead a life with far deeper human contact than most of us ever have, appealed very much to me.

'I suppose it was a road to Damascus kind of thing. I was visiting Europe and I went to see Findhorn. I liked the feel of it but I was cautious. I decided I would just stay a few days, but those days turned into months and then years. It was startling to find people really talking about what had gone on in their lives, wanting to know about me, and making me feel there was a place for me.

'I hadn't realized how lonely I had been until then and the sense of being cared about and having other people to care about in turn, has convinced me that, in some way or other, I want to live the rest of my life communally.'

George, who has been there some years and has set up a successful business making solar appliances which sell to the 'outside world', also feels Findhorn has been a place where he could 'grow up and learn to live with other people in a less egotistical way than I had done in my marriage'.

An interesting aspect of the Findhorn Foundation is that, although the Caddys were mature when they started it, their disciples tended to be much younger. But those who have stayed have, of course, aged so that these days there is a caucus of mid-lifers and some older than that, with many of these people regarding the community as home, the place where they will grow old. When I visited there was a growing awareness that the community has to look at what this means and how it will deal with an ageing population.

It is imperative that this should be done, in the view of Lucia who, at seventy-four, is one of the eight oldest residents in the Findhorn community. She left her home and work in San Francisco to come here twelve years ago, after reading several books about the place. She recalls a decision made on whim: 'I just thought this is it . . . I was living quite a solitary existence and without much sense of purpose. My marriage had ended, relations with my married daughter were difficult and I had begun to have a grim sense of marking time and being out of place in a society which seemed too much about materialism, too little about caring and sharing.'

She sits in the small room, her private domain in the erstwhile college building which is converted into residential units and rooms used for workshops and social gatherings, with its view down into a valley of trees. She is a smartly dressed, immaculately made-up woman whose style suggests a senior executive rather than the spiritual refugee style often associated with the Findhorn Foundation.

Her pleasure in life here, the sense she has of being usefully involved in the running of the place and of being amongst good friends, is the thing she says first and emphatically. But that said, and understood, she moves on to the issues around ageing which preoccupy her.

She explains: 'When I arrived here, as a sixty-two-year-old, coming into a society of mostly much younger people, I became aware that my age was seen as a problem. I'd never given it any particular thought up until then. I knew that this was a "working community" and that was one of the things that appealed to me because I had never considered retirement in any sense and nor have the other older people here. The point of living in a mixed generation society where everyone plays a part in running things, is that retirement doesn't have to exist as a concept.

'Not one of us older people came with the idea of being taken care of in mind. I came full of enthusiasm for starting a more active and adventurous life than I was living in America. It just didn't occur to me that AGE would be a block. But I found that, even here, they had taken on a value system which is so widespread in British society where age is seen as contagious and people don't really want to be associated with it.'

Such an attitude, she explains, seemed curiously out of place in a community built – and very successfully – on humanitarian and spiritual values, but Lucia says, 'I got a strong sense of the feeling that when you are sixty that's it, and that older people represented a problem.'

It was not something a woman as feisty as Lucia was going to quietly accept. She saw her first 'task' being to demonstrate that her age was not a disadvantage in any practical sense, and then to set about the 'political' aspect. She took on a range of jobs in administration, reception, at the in-house publishing company and now she is on the editorial board. She says, fiercely, that she works as hard as anybody and adds: 'As I settled in and saw that I, and the other older people, really are just as integrated, in every way, as the younger people whether through work, going to groups or in contributing our thoughts, ideas and experiences, I felt increasingly that it was important to tackle the ageism I saw. Partly it was important for me and my contemporaries but also for the community. The Findhorn Foundation talks of itself as open to anyone who wants to commit to its way of life, yet they haven't got to grips with the fact that people do age.'

It says something about the sense of security Lucia feels among people she describes as 'my very dear friends' and the fact that they are open to looking at issues and have a genuine desire to be democratic, that Lucia felt able to become, effectively, a one-woman anti-ageism campaign.

She explains: 'It was no use being angry or upset. Feelings about age are universal and the important thing is to go into battle over them, not just fade quietly or bitterly away. I think older people have a responsibility to prove to the youngsters that their prejudices may be wrong.'

So she has spent a good deal of time raising the issue, talking, tackling prejudices head-on when she sees them, and she talks of holding seminars where age will be the topic. 'For so long Findhorn had just young or youngish people, but that is changing. There are fears about older people getting ill and dying and the community doesn't have a strategy for coping with that so I think it is wary of older people. But it's no good having a community which doesn't acknowledge older people and I see myself as a pioneer working for change.

'I see the new ageing phenomenon, where we expect to have longer lives, as an adventure – an adventure I get to have first and I can tell others about it, so that should make me a valuable guide.'

A very different community is the Samye Ling Tibetan Meditation Centre which attracts older people who want a contemplative and tranquil environment and, in many cases, the opportunity to follow Tibetan teachings and to be amongst people with shared values.

The Centre opened more than a quarter of a century ago, after the Tibetans who founded it had fled from China and come to Britain. It was established as a religious centre, and the ornate, brightly coloured temple of worship they built can be glimpsed between the knitted brows of the dark pine trees. It has grown in the years to become a place where anyone wanting a retreat, to study Tibetan meditation or simply to find a quiet space, may come and stay for a few days or weeks.

A small group of people who see themselves as looking for a lifestyle away from materialistic values, or who have decided that they did not want to spend the whole of life caught in a career structure, living in the fast lane at whatever price, have made it their home. A few have come and stayed to take orders and become monks and nuns.

Among them are Gwen and Harry who have built their own house in the Centre grounds – something which is permitted if the building is donated to the Centre when the owners die.

Gwen is now in her sixties, Harry in his seventies – an age, Harry observes, with a certain satisfaction, when people seem to think they must wind down: 'It's not like that here. There's always so much to do – I'm an electrical engineer and some-one's always after me to help them with a project. Gwen and I are cut off from the main house and the flow of visitors for courses and short stays, and it's a relief because that's not our thing. But we certainly contribute to the running of the place, and people do plenty for us in return. We live amongst people who are close friends, with whom we share a philosophy, although nobody insists on that or expects us to have more to do with the faith than we want. I think it would be impossible to be miserable and alone here because someone would always check you out if you hadn't been around for a while.'

Gwen and Harry study the Tibetan faith, but also lead an ordinary domestic life, having their children and grandchildren to stay, inviting people for meals, visiting friends away from the Centre. Gwen looks back to their reasons for coming: 'The children had grown up, there was just the two of us. Harry had retired and I saw very clearly how easy it would be to just wind down, getting slower and slower and older and older because we weren't required to do anything, and cut off from a more vigorous community.

'We had visited Samye Ling often because we are both interested in Tibetan Buddhism and we felt more and more drawn to the idea of becoming involved in the place and making it our home for the rest of our lives. It means that if Harry dies before I do, which is probable, my life will go on. Of course it will be very sad, there will be grief, but I shall be among people I feel very close to and that must make a great difference.'

When I visited Braziers I felt an immediate affinity with the people there and it has lingered on in my mind as a place where I could imagine growing old. Sitting in the dishevelled sitting room talking with Margaret and Nonie, two of the core community, I felt very much at home, very much that it would be comfortable to quietly join in and let life drift on towards a mellow old age.

Braziers was started in 1952 by Glynn Faithfull, then approaching his forties, and separated from the mother of singer Marianne Faithfull. He decided he wanted to grow old living in a community and, not finding what he wanted already up and running, he set about founding Braziers in a beautiful Gothic stone house in fifty acres of Oxfordshire countryside which he and psychoanalyst Norman Glaister, who shared his vision, managed to acquire.

Since that time Braziers has grown and weathered, going through its share of troubles Glynn acknowledges, but these days it is a settled and optimistic place and in amongst a long and fascinating saga of how the place evolved, he talks of having a wonderfully invigorating and rewarding time as an elder. One of the things, it seems, that one inevitably sacrifices when living communally is a degree of autonomy – the trade-off presumably for the virtue of having a secure place in a close-knit society. At Braziers they have a room each in the main house, although one of the long-term members, a former British Rail worker in his sixties, who now works as the community's accountant, has a small house in the grounds. Otherwise the sitting room, dining room and study rooms are shared. Cooking is done on a rota and all meals are eaten together. It means upsets, unhappinesses and illness are quickly spotted, explains Glynn's wife Margaret, but it also imposes a degree of sociability which I suspect could get onerous at times. When and if the time comes that I design a communal lifestyle I shall avoid enforced gregariousness.

The fundamental community here is just a handful of men and women and all are aged over sixty. But foreign students coming to stay for a year or two, helping with the heavy work in return for board, young adults sometimes with children, and mid-lifers staying for indefinite times either paying their way or working at the upkeep of the place, create the feel of an animated mixed generation community. At weekends courses ranging from life-skills to the academic are held and these bring an influx of outsiders who may stay overnight, and even though the courses are kept well down in price, they are a vital part of Braziers' financing.

On the day I visited, early afternoon sunshine slanted through the arched windows of the dining hall, picking out the long table where lunch was being eaten. Just about every age group from a toddler in a buggy next to his young mum, through to the zesty, now eighty-one-year-old Glynn, was gathered, sharing food prepared and served by residents. Talk was animated and there was a good deal of laughter as Michael, a drama student in his thirties who had chosen this as home, flirted with sixty-four-year-old Margaret, Glynn's wife, while Nonie, a widow in her sixties who came to live at Braziers after her husband died, chided him for his impertinence.

In answer to a question about the problems of getting older she becomes quite fierce: 'Ageing – I wonder why folk dread it so. As long as one is fit, it doesn't have to be a problem – not anyway if one lives in a community.'

The mixing of generations brings different perspectives and attitudes, as happens at best in natural families and Margaret thinks this vital: 'The mix of generations is very important. We really do all learn from each other. I might just as easily ask Michael or Bruce, two young men who have been living here a while, their opinion on something, or for advice on how I might tackle a particular task, as they would ask me something they don't know. I suspect there are fewer tensions about this happening because we aren't natural family. A retirement community where you choose to be cut off from younger people seems a ghastly idea to me. Far from reminding us how old we are, the youngsters keep us aware of different ideas in the world, they are fun, they are active and they do seem to pay some deference to our years. The nicest thing is that friendship develops quite naturally between the generations.'

But of course there are discordant times; problems, anger and coping with this, finding resolution which is essential if the community is to survive, can be hard going Glynn acknowledges, but it is also, he insists, a constructive process because people learn not to simply withdraw from each other when things are uncomfortable but to listen to each other's viewpoints, understand why they may be different from their own and reach some kind of reconciliation. This process is formalized in a weekly meeting when everyone comes together and has an opportunity to talk about how they are feeling about life in the community, to air grievances, to bring before the others disagreements or rows which have erupted between individuals. Glynn explains: 'The important thing about these meetings is that everybody knows what they have to say will be heard. The meeting is structured with someone guiding it, so whereas a group of individuals might interrupt each other and just get angry, the person in charge has to make sure this doesn't happen and that everybody gets the opportunity to explain their position properly. It also allows people to talk out the kind of feelings of insecurity, unhappiness with the way they are being treated, all that sort of thing. We consider this meeting an important part of our life together because it really is about growing constantly and refining the business of living together.'

Then, reflecting on this post-war dream of creating a lifestyle for what he describes as 'constructive ageing' Glynn says: 'The thing that, fundamentally, makes Braziers work is the involvement we have with each other and the sense of purpose about what we are doing.

'Keeping the place going involves daily work and that is the responsibility of everyone who is not too old or too young to be physically up to it. We all value Braziers and get a lot out of living in such a lovely place so there is a commitment there which binds us. It also means we are not sitting around wondering what to do with ourselves feeling neglected and lost as, sadly, old people too often end up doing.'

Given how much most of us worry about the circumstances in which we will die, one of the most appealing and reassuring things about the communities I visited, is the unquestioning way in which they care for anyone ill or dying. At Samye Ling they talked of the last days of one of their members. Ani Lodrho who lives there told me: 'We just sat with him at the end and, because we believe in re-incarnation, we talked about the journey he was going on and what he had meant to us in this life. We kept chatting and joking and he joined in. Then, quite quietly, he died. We held a service for him with lots of flowers and prayers – it was very beautiful and his spirit is still here, very much so.'

Margaret, too, described the recent death of a woman who had been a long-term member of the Braziers group: 'She was ill for a while, and we made sure there was always someone there once she became bed-ridden. In the last days, when it was clear she was dying, those of us who were really close to her, sat around her bed and just stayed with her until she died. I can think of nothing worse than being alone at that time.'

When people are in couples they may value separateness and their own routine, over-involvement with others, but for single people, who reach mid-life and fear growing old alone the appeal is very clear. A new home cannot in itself fill the gap left when children go or the regret when there have been no children, or wipe away the pain left by a partner who has died or gone, but taking on a new way of living can certainly act as a palliative. And joining an active communal household could be the thing that helps us to see the future as an adventure not an endurance test.

Susan, who is approaching fifty and is on her own and childless, regularly visited a long-established community where friends lived, during her childhood, and she is clear: 'It is probably what I will choose. I compare the kind of future I am likely to have on my own – I already suffer a lot of loneliness – with the animation of the community. There's always something going on there – activities being organized, gardens to be looked after and there's quite a lot of involvement with the village outside. Of course there's a downside: people don't always get on, there are sometimes rows and problems, and of course you are involved in those as part of the community, and I can see this might be tiresome. But I consider that a lot better than the kind of fading out I see in lonely old people.'

These communities, which are about people coming together to create a common lifestyle, strive to make it possible for those who want to join to do so. At Findhorn people can earn their keep; at Braziers those with some income are generally asked to contribute, but there are also 'allowance' situations as Glynn put it. A retired or redundant person is as eligible as any other provided they do their share of community work.

The quest for a community where fundamental ideals are shared is, in the view of Professor Otto van Mering, Director of the Centre for Gerontological Studies at the University of Florida, an optimistic belief in the future by the ageing population. He says: 'People are creating communities to re-discover their own worth, survivability and maybe even their soul. Ironically it is not the young but the *old* in their retirement years who are seeking Utopian community living.'

The kinds of communities described here, and those which van Mering talks of where the accommodation may have been set up with ageing people in mind and with health care on site, but where the inhabitants are involved in activities – running the library, setting up courses, outings, or else going into the outside community to work as volunteers – seem to me a healthy alternative to isolation and the sense of futility we hear all too much about. The advantages to these custom-created centres is that they have facilities and health workers living there so one of the fears we face as we age – that we may have an accident or be taken ill and have nobody to call on – is not a worry, but other than that independence is encouraged and the emphasis is very much on continuing to be a contributing and involved member of society.

By contrast the Florida and California-style mega-retirement communities, where fun-fun-fun until you drop seems to be the guiding principle, and where a huge range of activities, sports, entertainment is laid on, seem to me deeply paternalis-tic. Beth Wood whose mother has lived in a retirement village in Florida for some years describes how: 'The staff talk to the inhabitants as though they are small children who need to be humoured and the activities echo that. They are all about providing jolly things to do so the people never stop and think about the fact that they are ageing. I consider it unhealthy. I'd far rather see my mother being a straightforward old woman and being able to accept that because I think she would be happier than rushing off to join in seniors' bathing belle contests and other such nonsense.'

These retirement communities are effectively mini-worlds with their own shops, hairdressers, restaurants, and a huge range of activities and entertainments, and residents are often tagged with such euphemisms as young-elderly. Within these ghettos, which usually have a lower age limit of fifty, the idea appears to be that if we isolate ourselves we can also fool ourselves we are not old at all and play blithely at the 'I'm as young as I feel' game; we can escape from a world where youth might rear its gorgeous head reminding us that this is what we cannot have.

At first glimpse such places may be very beguiling and, as retirement is a stage which tells us very clearly that we have reached the end of the major goal-oriented part of our life, so it is understandable that people may want to be given an alternative lifestyle to enter into.

But it seems to me we should pause and consider carefully the implications of such places which are not about ideology so much as about commerce and profit and there must be a vested interest in creating dependency.

What people buy in these 'active retirement' homes – these big and profitable businesses in which, to secure a place, people must start saving or take out an insurance policy almost with the first wrinkle – is cosseting. It seems to me that what we are choosing if we go into such an environment is the chance to be infantilized, to give up responsibility for being a grown-up who can cope with the real world and all its challenges.

And the sad truth is that handing oneself over rather than striving to take responsibility for ourselves, leaves us open to exploitation and cruelty. Journalist Richard Grant revealed a chilling lack of compassion or care when he visited one retirement community in California and found the community turning like a pack of wolves on those who become sick and are clearly dying, insisting they be removed from the community. Grant saw in what happened a profound fear of death, the recognition that no matter how merrily you skid off in motorized caddies around the golf courses, no matter how hip the dancing at the disco nights, we are ultimately all ageing and we will die. So, rather than finding a way of sharing the fears and dealing with them, these communities go into hectic denial. But isn't that kind of denial ultimately the loneliest and most scary state of all?

The contrast with the approach of Samye Ling or Braziers to illness and death is stark indeed.

And surely if we live among other people part of the point is that we care for each other. At best this happens in ways described here, in communal situations. It also happens in other circumstances where people are integrated with each other and bonds have formed, but if we want to create that situation as individuals we may need to think carefully about how it can be done.

Maud, who is widowed, chose to remain in the small seaside town where she had brought up her children, even though she needed to sell the family house once they had gone, and even though it meant living far from her grandchildren. Claudia, her daughter, now in her late forties, sees how wise a choice this was: 'If Mum had come to London she would have been at a loose end and probably rather lost. I couldn't have spent enough time with her to fill all the gaps which would have been left in her life. She has a very active social life and is a stalwart of the community, doing volunteer work, helping to organize local events and offering board and lodging for musicians when they come to perform in the annual festival.

'We visit her regularly, which is lovely, and she's never bored. It's been the perfect way for her. She is a very private person and needs to be able to shut her door and do things her own way, but I also know people are around enough that if she becomes ill there will be someone there immediately. She's in her eighties now and frail so I visit frequently and I'm on the phone a lot. We have plenty of contact. I look to the way she has done things and think how wise she was to make a decision about how she would live while she was still middle-aged so that it has carried on and she has made friends among other people who planned in the same way, to live out their lives in the town.

'It is wonderful for me, too, because I know that if she's ill there are friends who will make sure she's all right, and if something happened to Mum there would be plenty of people around immediately doing whatever needed doing. I don't think being alone is at all worrying for her.'

Living in a small, caring community is every bit as important for American Charlie Fox who, although only in his fifties, has multiple sclerosis throughout his body, so that his head is the only thing he can still move. Here he is among people who have watched his illness progress, and who continue to think of him as, in the words of one neighbour, 'one of the brightest, funniest, most bolshie people you could imagine'. Charlie is a character, somebody people enjoy visiting because he is a great conversationalist, very well read, and it would be hard to regard him as a suitable case for too much sympathy. He has a day-time carer but every evening a local friend pops in to make sure he is all right, as they do first thing in the morning. Looking out over a lake full of tall still reeds, caught in the fading afternoon light, Charlie sees his lot as very similar to that of an incapacitated older person: 'I can't *do* much but I can be a good friend, have a joke, make interesting conversation. People seem to enjoy coming to see me and I feel very much part of my neighbourhood.'

The majority of people choose to live as Maud does, alone, but for many of us there is the worry that we will become dependent on our children. Tom, a divorced father of three, voices the concern of many mid-lifers, who have grappled with the problems of dependent parents: 'I don't want my kids to feel they should look after me in later life. I don't want them to feel they can't live abroad or to feel guilty all the time wondering if I'm festering away all on my own waiting for them to visit. I know that feeling only too well from my own family – it wasn't their fault but my parents lived in an area where all their close friends seemed to have left and they just seemed to live for my visits. I am an active person at present and I am absolutely determined that I'll keep up being that or I'll move in with other people – whatever, I am determined to keep up a busy lifestyle. Then my kids coming around would be a bonus but not a lifeline.'

Many of the schemes described here have evolved at least in part as a substitute for life in an extended family or among a mix of generations in the neighbourhood. Howard, a forty-year-old American sometime actor and taxi driver who lives and works in the hilly Marin County region of California, talks of how the community where he lives has come to recognize the loss of a generation of elders who have an interest and emotional investment in the younger generations.

He lives in a group which set out to be self-sufficient and did not pay enough attention to family roots in its youthful, ideological quest for a place where members could build an alternative lifestyle. He explains: 'People came from different parts of the world – Europe, Australia, the big American cities – and that gave us a kind of unity, a sense of being very self-sufficient. But there was almost a complete loss of family. There were some older people but virtually nobody had their parents around. It was when the younger people began coupling up and having children that they became very aware of what a loss it is not to have parents and grandparents around.'

They saw very clearly how their children needed someone who knew more than they do about the world. There was quite a lot of sadness and Howard explains: 'Out of that grew the idea that we could ask the older people who are here to become surrogate grandparents and in some cases they have moved into the homes where families live. They are given free accommodation and food and in return they take the role of a grandparent involving themselves with the children, helping care for them, and being there as a source of knowledge and experience.

'The older people know that when they become frail and need help their "family" will be there. In Bolinas old people are at a premium and families have to compete to "win" one!'

The pleasure young and old generations can get from mixing and learning from each other has been much battered in the post-war era where the idea of youth rebelling against the elderly, and older people becoming hostile curmudgeons in the face of youth culture has become established as the way things are. Yet although the Giles cartoon of the granny waving her umbrella at a scruffy young thing, makes for entertainment, it is a misrepresentation which quite clearly adds to polarization and discrimination. In truth, older people when surveyed stated very firmly that they enjoy the company of the young, and many dislike very much the idea of being segregated from them.

Yet that is exactly what happens to many grandparents who find they are far from their children and grandchildren so that visiting is difficult. And as many of us know, however keen we are for our children to see their grandparents, making a long journey regularly, in an anyway busy work schedule, can put a lot of strain on relations. Jane Blair expresses it: 'My kids adore Mum and Dad and it's important for them to see each other – I very much want them to have a close relationship. But my partner and I both work and frankly at the weekends we want to just potter with the kids. But once a month we do go and stay with one or other of our parents, but it's far from an ideal way of keeping contact.'

For Lucy Darwall-Smith, her husband Philip and their daughter Daisy, the perfect solution, as they laughingly say it, has been: 'Putting Gran in the attic upstairs!' Anne Eade, who lives in a granny flat at the top of their house knew well the problems which can arise when a parent lives with children and, keen though she was to be close to her own daughter and her grandchild, she was wary when her daughter first suggested that she move in.

She feared becoming a burden and says, quite fiercely, 'I looked after my own mother until she died at ninety-three and although she was a terrific character and we had always got on very well, it was a huge strain and effort in the last years. I really don't want to think this is what Lucy would have to cope with.' Lucy, who has a demanding job and 'absolutely no free time' appreciated this and she acknowledges: 'My mother is wonderful at present, she's a terrific Granny for Daisy who adores her, and she's a real help to me because she's there if I'm out and Daisy can go up and visit.

'She'll babysit, she's always willing to help out and I know she likes to do that.

'But I wouldn't want to give everything up to look after Mummy if she got ill, and she has said very firmly that she doesn't want me to do that. So we're putting money aside to pay for help if that happens. That way she can be cared for here, we'll be able to be around and see plenty of her. And none of us has to worry about her becoming a burden.'

Before Anne moved in there were some lengthy round-table discussions, during which an agreement was drawn up on what everybody wanted and expected out of the arrangement, and what they all thought important as boundaries.

Lucy is very clear that this is essential: 'It seems important that you are all on the same wavelength and that the granny flat thing be arranged so that it is not seen as living together but as a way of being close and companionable while living separately. It means we see each other on a daily basis but we can also choose not see each other if that is how we feel. We talked a good deal about how much we should be family. For instance I quite often take Mum a plate of what I've cooked for supper, but the assumption is that she cooks for herself unless I offer something. She looks after her own place, has her own social life and she has her part of the garden to tend. She has a standing invitation to Sunday lunch and I often invite her down for a drink early evening.

'But the fact that it is an invitation not a right is all-important to establish. I've seen these arrangements become utter hell because the old person either thinks they can be part of everything and the couple has no privacy, or they need endless reassurance that they are loved and that is a huge strain. I don't think setting these things up is easy but I think it could be successful far more often if people laid out the ground rules first.'

Anne has taken out continuing power of attorney for Lucy and Philip so that, no matter what happens to her mental abilities, they will be able to manage her affairs. But for now she is a vigorous, droll seventy-eight-year-old who gardens long and hard and will then be visited more often than not by granddaughter Daisy at tea-time. Anne laughs now at the anxieties she had before moving and says, 'I regard this as being the happiest time of my life. If I can live like this until the end I'll feel I've had a good run.'

Mary Windsor, in her fifties, is now grandmother to five. She moved to northern Scotland, close to two of her children both with partners, so that she could be part of her grandchildren's daily lives. She has no wish to live with either family, but has a tiny, wind-blown pre-fab where she revels in her independence and the quiet in which to write stories, poetry and journalism. She explains: 'I was very clear that I wanted to be part of the kids' lives, I didn't want to be the distant granny and the arrangement I have seems the best possible. I get huge pleasure from the grandchildren, watching them grow, hearing their ideas on life, meeting their friends and they are interested in what I do too. The relationship I have with my own children has improved a great deal because I'm around but not in charge of them. I'm an adult friend.'

Bringing people into one's own house may be another way of offsetting loneliness. Betty Saltiel, who is widowed, found that her house seemed echoey and too empty after her husband died, but she did not want the commitment of setting up home with other people. She says: 'I have got used to living alone and I value my space and privacy. I have lodgers periodically, sometimes from the local theatre when they are there performing, which is always entertaining. At the moment I have a student.' Anna Kemp, too, has taken in students since she was divorced and although she lays down very clear rules to begin with about what is and is not allowed – for instance times for using the kitchen – if she becomes friendly with a student these rules are often relaxed. She enjoys very much a role which makes her 'part parent to a younger person who is often alone in the country, and part friend. I get quite involved with the lives of the students, sometimes, when we become friendly, and I like to think they value the fact that I am a bit older and more worldly than they are. With some I've gone to cinemas and theatres or on outings with them. I started taking in students after the divorce and I realized I was dreading going home from work to an empty house.'

Of course many people do not own their own homes and mid-life is none too soon to take a look at what may be on offer if we have to move as we age. A valuable first step is to look at successful state housing schemes where people seem to live contentedly, and find out whether something similar could be created in our own areas. But getting local authorities to be responsive to their constituents' needs is not always easy and we would do well to start campaigning to make housing a far more potent political issue than it is at present.

Leading gerontologists in the US liken the impact the current demographic changes will have on society and the scale of the challenge it poses for social policy to the Industrial Revolution. Jane Porcino, author of *Living Longer, Living Better: Adventures in Community Housing for Those in the Second Half of Life* believes it is essential that housing be pushed 'to the top of the national agenda'.

The important thing is not to demand just housing, but to make sure we are sufficiently involved in the planning and development process to be able to design a lifestyle that we want. A fine example of this process was Bradeley Village, an independent community for 240 over-fifty-five-year-olds near Stoke-on-Trent in the North of England.

The idea for it came from Amsterdam's HBB housing association and it is sufficiently successful that requests for something similar are being heard from around the country. Alongside the streets of houses are shops, meeting places, several leafy open spaces all under cover. Journalist Michael Simmons, no youngster himself, wrote of this village in the *Guardian* with the kind of enthusiasm which suggests he might like to be slipped on to the waiting list:

Walking today through the main entrance, an airy, hotel-like 'buzz' is immediately apparent. Tenants sit about in small groups, in armchairs at brightly coloured tables, drinking coffee, served at thirty-five pence a cup from the resident-run counter. The reception desk is also the village's management and security office from which everyone entering through the (automatic) front door is screened.

Before designing the homes and facilities the Housing Association consulted with potential residents at a series of public meetings which also got everyone talking, sharing views, listening to each other's reasons for their wishes, and it turned out that more than half the people wanting to live there also wanted to be involved in running the village.

They chose to have a grocer's shop which they would run on a co-op basis, a library, a laundry, licensed bar as well as a social club with dancing and bingo and all are now being run by residents. Some, explains Simmons, are earning revenue which will be ploughed back into producing further amenities and outings.

One reason other councils might avert their eyes from this obvious example to follow would be fear of it being too costly but this has not been the case with Bradeley Village. Residents pay moderate rents and there are already plans for another village to be built along the same lines. This project evolved from a belief that older people deserve decent housing and the word the Association team who worked with residents use is 'dignity' for their community.

Creating the 'intimacy and distance' which was how elderly people interviewed by a team of German researchers described their ideal, preoccupied architect John Melvin when he was asked to create a sheltered housing scheme for residents in north London inside the façade of a row of houses. His idea, which won a design award and also appears to have achieved a *modus operandi* which makes for happy tenants, is designed to have 'a collegiate feel' to it.

There is a lot of carved wood, panelling, and swirling varnished wooden banisters – it is an environment in which history and age are made to seem important. Melvin was determined there would be no institutional corridors so three blocks of flats are interlinked and flats have some distance from each other. One of the most appreciated features is a spare bedroom so friends and family can come to stay. There is a considerable sense of privacy but also a communal room where activities and events take place. A vision of such a place, where a sense of safety – there is a twenty-four-hour warden on duty – goes cheek by jowl with the chance to be 'an eccentric old misfit when I feel like it' is how Jenny, now in her late forties, envisages living: 'I quite like the idea of sheltered housing, not having responsibility for running the show, but privacy – that's important. I don't think I'd mind living alone and I like the idea there might be entertainment laid on – but I hope it won't be Victorian music hall by my time!'

In this chapter I have set out to explore some of the living schemes which appear to be better alternatives to the isolation and loneliness which too many people talk of as they get older. They differ in style but the thing they have in common is that residents feel they are part of a society where it is implicit that people care for each other and it is that sense which has been lost in our society. But not everyone wants to move to a community or set up a home with others, and so it is that communitarianism has become the buzz concept of the moment. This basically means breaking with the individualism which has made us assiduously avoid too much intimacy with neighbours and creating closer bonds with and taking responsibility for what goes on within our community.

Not Mellow But Outraged

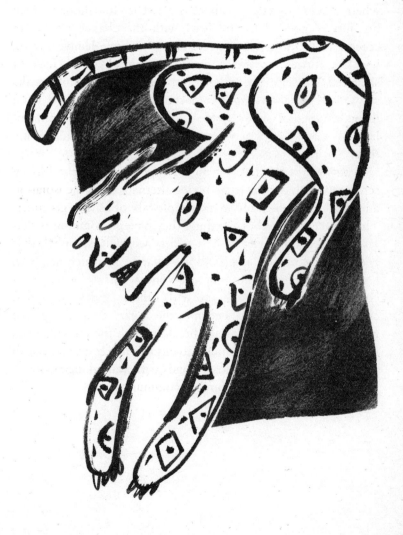

> I will never be an old man. To me old age is always
> fifteen years older than I am.
>
> BRENDAN BARUCH

'A PLAGUE OF WRINKLIES' was the jokey lead in to a commentary in the *Guardian* newspaper, discussing what the so-called grey boom will mean for governments as they have to provide for ever-growing numbers of elderly people. 'Age race wars' howled the American press, in headlines which conjure a picture of the young and the old slugging it out on the streets. What they were actually suggesting is that children will be deprived because of the cost in the future of caring for the elderly's needs. And what about 'pension snatchers' and 'benefit bandits', nice little terms I have heard used in discussions about the amounts already being paid out? Do we take it that our elders have been assailing Securicor vans transporting pensions, or kitting themselves out with handkerchief scarves over nose and mouth, guns at the ready?

Not exactly. What we are witnessing is a crude and cruel kind of attrition directed towards our elders who are, by implication, being blamed for the fact they are the fastest growing group in the population, and for having the temerity, thanks to a better standard of living and health care, to live longer, thus confronting governments with the taxing problem of how to look after them. Where in all this is the belief that older people, who have spent their lives working to support and care for younger generations, should be rewarded with care and support in their later years? It is a peculiarly shameful product of the past couple of decades that the notion of a society caring for its own when they are least able to do so for themselves – a philosophy made policy in Britain with Beveridge's welfare state after the last war – has been so rubbished. No wonder Maggie Kuhn, seventy-five-year-old leader of the Grey Panthers, the American militant group for the elderly, greets the world with an embattled expression and says unequivocally: 'We're not mellowed, sweet old people. We're outraged, but we're doing something about it.'

As mid-lifers we may applaud such feisty sentiments but see them as little to do with us. We have problems of our own grappling with the middle years, so that time beyond seems somehow remote. But we would be wise to stop and re-consider this perspective, partly because the lack of humanity being dished out to older people is not something we should tolerate, but also for ourselves and our futures. It is unlikely there will be a sudden volte-face in attitudes as we become elders unless we start taking the way elders are treated seriously right now, tackling everything from demeaning language and treatment of older people, to outright discrimination.

We know well how damaging racism and sexism are – can you imagine talking about a plague of blacks or women? And ageism is widespread as we hear from the authors of the Eurobarometer Survey who have found 'age discrimination in all member states'. Nor does ageism have an official starting time, and even though its full impact will probably be felt most by the eldest it will surely filter into our lives in many different ways during the middle years. We may not see issues of resources and pensions for example, as an immediate concern, but we are certainly affected by the attitudes of a society which wants young over old any day.

Jenny Knight says: 'I am coming up for fifty and I am very aware of the different ways in which people react to the ageing or aged. One is to ignore them and to assume that they no longer have any valuable social contribution to make. Another is to see them as helpless. I'm not there yet but I see it around me and I become increasingly aware that this is what I can expect if things don't change.' Gordon Bloom, in his late fifties, is daunted by 'the absolute lack of interest I see in issues which affect the elderly. If their pensions are cut, fuel taxed, if they die of hypothermia in winter, the stories get nothing like the prominence or attention they would if we were talking about the young having a tough time. And a story about an old person doing something remarkable will get half an inch compared to some drivel about a sexy-looking young woman doing nothing in particular.'

Alice Jones was startled to find ageist attitudes in a world she had assumed would value her life's experience so far. She says, 'I hardly consider fifty old but was told it was too old for a university career. Similarly I have been trying to get accepted to train as a Jungian analyst, but in England there is a fifty- to fifty-five-year-old cut-off point. Amazing at an age when I'm just beginning to find some wisdom.'

Ageism may be more pernicious than other discriminations because it is wrapped in the double bind of sentimental myth delighting in the stereotypes of rosy-cosy sweet old dears and salts of the earth, while in reality old people pose problems society does not want to engage in, its resentment coming out in all sorts of forms. In the paper 'Ageing in Society' the authors put it this way: 'Images of ageing are often ambivalent. On the one hand they express concern for the old and frail whilst on the other they reveal anxiety and even fear. The disturbing image of old age as a dirty secret of decrepit sub-human beings on the edge of death, who can only be physically and mentally shut away, will be difficult to displace from centre-stage.'

It is in the workplace that we are most likely, in the middle years, to be made to realize that age, far from being seen as a reason why we may have knowledge, expertise and confidence in our work, is a disadvantage. Work is the one place where discrimination is still openly permitted and job advertisements regularly state an upper age limit – often below forty and rarely above. In a report 'Ageing – Why Fight it?' commissioned by Collagen UK Ltd, a company marketing anti-ageing treatments, a spot check on job ads for office workers in *The Times* on one day in 1994 was described. There were 169 vacancies and only one ad stated 'no age restrictions'. The Carnegie Inquiry into the Third Age looked into employment possibilities for the over-fifties and concluded that many people are never given a chance to demonstrate whether they are capable or not. Employers, they said, screen out older workers when recruiting. Older employees are refused the training and promotion opportunities offered to younger colleagues. The dismal ramification of this is that employers begin to believe older workers have lost the qualities they see as ideal. A survey of 500 personnel directors and employees throughout Britain, and of 1000 job applicants, carried out by Gallup Poll for Brook Street (1990) showed that more than three quarters of employers regard the under-thirty-fives as being most appropriate to meet their recruitment needs because 'younger workers are not set in their ways, are quicker thinking and have a grasp of modern technology'. Four in five employees believe they have been turned down for jobs because they were too old, even though they had the right skills.

Two Eurobarometer surveys were conducted in twelve member states to gauge public attitude towards ageing and older people. They were sponsored by the European Community and published in 1993. 'An extraordinarily high proportion of citizens in all EC countries were found to believe that older workers are discriminated against when it comes to job promotion and training', and fifteen- to twenty-four-year-olds were almost as likely to say this as those of forty-five plus.

Richard Worsley, director of the Carnegie Inquiry, observed something similar: 'Age discrimination is very widespread. Recruiters seem to think they will score Brownie points with employers if they come up with a lot of bright young things.'

Greg Lamb, an executive with a computer firm, knows about this: 'I'm in my mid-fifties and several younger people in the company were being sent on development courses. I asked if I could go too because I felt it would be valuable to learn about the most up-to-date approaches, but my boss as good as said it would be a waste of time and money.'

Valerie Simons watched a young woman brought in as her assistant promoted over her within eighteen months: 'I'm in my forties and, even though I say it myself, good at my job. I was brought in to sort out the extremely messy system of docketing and applying for payments which the firm had, and I succeeded so well that they were getting a consistently higher amount of money coming in each month. I was praised for that and for training the new assistant when she came. But I watched it happening: she is young, confident and she just targeted the boss and convinced him that she could be trained to be someone very valuable in the company. I could have been too, but I know they felt that's not what you do with a woman in her forties. It made me very upset.'

Jim, also in his mid-forties, found that: 'Younger chaps were being promoted over me at the insurance company where I work, even though I have far more knowledge and understanding of policies and how they will affect people, than a lot of these kids who may have been with us just a few years.'

As mid-lifers, then, we are directly in the firing line of this brand of ageism, which writes people off at an age when those promoting the rewards of middle age talk of this stage being the prime of life. The perceptions which lead to such treatment were spelled out by the Birmingham Settlement, a group set up in that town to look at issues affecting local people in a number of ways. One of their projects was to identify issues around mid-life and, until 1994, when it was cut, council funding was given for them to run workshops and groups to advise and help those feeling in need of this. Summing up the findings of their research they listed as 'Some myths about older workers' (compared with younger workers):

They are slower and less productive.
They are less creative.
They cannot cope with change.

They have high levels of absenteeism due to ill health.
They are not worth investing in.

The Settlement, drawing on the Local Government Board report for 1990, countered this with 'Some facts about older workers':

Surveys show absenteeism to be lower for older workers
– this has also been found in America.
People over fifty often have a higher output than younger
colleagues, due to experience, maturity and strong
work ethic.
A recent study of Open University graduates found that
students aged sixty to sixty-five did better in their results
than any other group.
In today's economic climate most people have experienced
great changes, older workers included.

What we are up against is employers' belief that employing the young is a sign of their progressiveness, their ability to spot winners, their youthful image. They have appointed ever younger people to key jobs, pushing them up the hierarchy, delighting in being picked out as having the youngest-ever company chairman, managing director, head of department or whatever. When Alan Rusbridger was appointed editor of the *Guardian* newspaper at the age of forty-one, there was just about as much breathless comment about the fact that as one columnist quipped 'he looks ten and a half' as that he was an exceptionally bright and able journalist.

We should not be surprised at such attitudes which stem from the post-war knee-jerk belief that being young is to be, per se, better than someone older no matter what skills are required. And the irony is that people are being dismissed, frozen out or never given a chance to prove themselves at ages which would once have been seen as still formative time, the age and stage where youngsters are learning and making mistakes – processes they need to go through before being given the reins. But these days we have TV chiefs, account executives, key media interviewers, stockbrokers in the city, top managers in business, often still in their thirties or even twenties. There are top politicians scarcely at mid-life. In all these categories there is a clear case for arguing that the advantages of the elder statesman who has gained more experience and *savoir faire* are obvious. So by the time you have reached mid-life you have either done it all and where do you go, or you haven't done it all and, because others younger are doing so, you have become dead wood. That is the bleakest scenario and of course it is not an invariable one: there are in every profession esteemed and valued older people whose expertise certainly is valued, but they tend either to own the companies or be the exceptions. Reflecting on some of the extremely talented, interesting people I worked with when younger, I see too many who, simply because they are seen to have been around too long, are back-watered to make space for new young names. Stephen Ward at the Equal Opportunities Commission Institute of Personnel Development who sees day after day the impact of discrimination inveighs against it as 'irrational, illogical and damaging'.

Sally Brook, a forty-something writer on a national newspaper respected for its gravitas, notes the paradox: 'The paper is looked to for the depth and integrity of what it says, and true there are a few older people writing leading articles, but the editor really has a passion for new young "finds" – young men in flowery shirts straight out of Oxbridge and still emotional children, or young women spotted because they can turn a streetwise phrase and will make the paper seem in touch with a young world. At the same time some of the men and women who have given years of their life to the paper, who are very bright and able with maturity of thought, get treated so shabbily that they cannot fail to know how little is thought of them even though theirs are the by-lines which were once highly respected.'

The idea that older workers are ossified, failing and incapable of keeping up with technological development is not borne out when we look around at science, academia, mathematics, architecture, catering, skilled manual labour, to name just a few areas of work where older people are functioning at a highly competent and competitive level. In many countries politicians are voted in after they have passed retirement age while, absurdly, the House of Commons in Britain voted out an anti age discrimination bill – even though a large number of people casting their votes would not have been there if age discrimination applied in politics. Equally it is paradoxical that many directors and company chiefs, who remain *in situ* into their seventies, will not keep employees to the same age, although an article in *Business* magazine patted on the back eighty-four-year-old Lord Forte, whose empire has no compulsory retirement age.

Men certainly feel acutely the pressure of the young blood behind them, the sense of their own built-in obsolescence, yet it appears that the reality of ageism at work is greater for women than for men. A Brook Street survey found that two people in five believed a woman with the same skills as a man was more likely to be discriminated against on grounds of age and a study of employers' attitudes to older workers recorded employers who considered women returning to work aged thirty-five as old. Christine Bailey, then thirty-six, was told by several agencies that it wasn't worth putting her name forward for jobs because she was too old, although to their credit the computer firm Compel took her on and at the age of forty-nine she won the *Business Pages* Executive PA of the year award. In a lengthy article for the *Observer* Charlotte Eager reported a number of examples of women with impressive skills applying for jobs which, ostensibly, required these and not even being given the time of day because they had topped forty, or hearing a horrified voice at the end of the line tell them there was no point in applying.

Not being able to get a job or being offered 'early retirement' around fifty in a tone of voice which suggests little choice, is an all too frequent occurrence. The prospect of enforced retirement is described by Alan Walker, Professor of Social Policy at the University of Sheffield, as 'the blunt brutality of age-barrier retirement', which he sees as being inappropriate and outmoded at a time when people expect to live longer and when they are quite clearly remaining competent for a decade or so after a retirement age fixed to suit a different era. He says, 'The system of retirement, solving a number of burning issues a century ago, has increasingly become a labour market mechanism which creates structured social disintegration of people of sixty and over, sometimes even fifty and over ... smaller and smaller proportions of [older] people participate in the workforce, so increasing numbers of them are not socially integrated in one of the most important areas of life.'

Not all of us, of course, wish to work beyond the retirement age and, provided we have the means to lead the life we wish, there are good reasons why we may choose to use the next stretch of life in different pursuits. Indeed the French refer to the so-named Third Age – fifty to seventy-five – as the 'age of living', the time which follows the age of work. Yet nearly two-fifths of all Europeans (Eurobarometer), said they wanted to continue working, while more than half would have liked to continue working part-time.

Malcolm Marcus is fifty-five and expresses a fear many of us feel of the time when he must stop working: 'I'm in marketing and I love the work, the constant stimulus, meeting new people, and the challenge of having to work out some difficult concepts. I know I'm good at it and I work well under a certain amount of pressure. I absolutely dread the idea of this part of life simply vanishing. I just see a terrible oasis of time and a feeling that I'll be bloody useless pottering in the garden or feeling I ought to take up hang-gliding. It all depresses me enormously.'

Rose Mitchell, who has worked as a supermarket cashier while her children were growing up, says: 'I like the discipline of coming to work. I have good friends here and I'd feel the draught all right without the money. But I'd be happy to cut down to, say, three days a week.' She speaks for many mid-lifers who could afford to work less once children have left home, mortgages are paid off – or almost – and where time for the things there are never time for in earlier life, would be welcomed.

But this is not the solution for everybody, and there is something particularly cruel about forcing people out of work and into financial anxiety at an age at which we can now expect to be only halfway through life.

For Bill, in his mid-fifties, the worry is money: 'I haven't been able to save much but we've managed okay with my salary coming in regularly and my wife sometimes doing a bit of part-time work. But I don't know how we'll manage when I'm finished. I'm fit enough, likely to last a good few years, but it'll be tough on just the state money and I don't look forward to retirement.'

The prospect of so many people, younger in mind and body than generations before have been, equipped with the best of the post-war education and motivation, skilled through years of working in environments where innovation has been constant, being shown the door as they pass sixty-five and no argument, is drawing uncomfortably close in the lives of the post-war generations. The erstwhile acceptance of a set-age, inflexible retirement is beginning to be challenged. This challenge has come in the form of approaches to government, outspoken writings, and the spread of ideas through the media by the campaigning Carnegie Inquiry, the authors of *The Time of Our Life – Employment and Retirement in the Third Age* and the authors of *Is Retirement Working?* published by the Re-Action Trust, a joint initiative of British Industry and Help the Aged. These efforts take us in the right direction, but it is also up to us, today's mid-lifers, to take on the issue and put effort into re-casting ideas on older workers as well as looking at ways work might be re-structured.

One way would be for the working day – Britain has the longest in Europe – to be made shorter, thus easing up some of the strains on families with growing children and creating work which older people could take on. The advantage to this approach is that it would enable older people to have work without preventing the young from getting their opportunities.

Other ideas now being floated by those looking at ways forward are part-time work, a phase-out period for those who want it and preparation for retirement to help people re-think and re-structure their lives after work. The Carnegie Inquiry is urging employers' organizations to get rid of all age-related criteria where there is no absolute justification for it, to focus on why it might be a good thing to start looking at the potential of older workers and to offer them training. And while they are about it they might outlaw books like *How to Start A New Career* by Judith Johnstone which eulogizes about the qualities in workers up to forty then lists the over-forty-year-old as 'not nearly as ambitious as you were, possibly planning for early retirement, much less energetic or innovative, difficult to retrain'.

The Carnegie Inquiry also asks trade unions to promote policies which will help with flexible retirement and pensions. The Association of Retired Persons, an all-party pressure group lobbying for reforms to benefit older people, has backed this. Robert Rose, a retired businessman and chairman of ARP, asks: 'If you are seventy-five and doing the job well, why shouldn't you go on working?'

Why not indeed? But it is not enough for us simply to applaud such gestures. If we want these matters to be taken seriously, to be heard as the voice of a substantial part of the nation, we must each individually put in our protests and our requests, join organizations, sign petitions, dream up strategies for change. It is not just a question of the feelgood factor. If we are going to live longer than ever before – and gerontologists are talking about a hundredth birthday becoming commonplace – then we will need the means to support ourselves. The anguished contortions of governments across Europe and America, contemplating the cost of caring for the elderly might be eased if, as we get older but not less able, we were helped to help ourselves.

There are certainly ways this could be done, but it would require radicalism and bravery on the part of governments. There are plenty of kinds of work which need doing and for which older people would be very appropriate – in the environment, working with children. Age Concern are setting up a scheme whereby older people will work with children with special needs for example, and in schools extra help in the classroom is often badly needed. Older people can work well in youth clubs and organizing activities. They could be employed to train newcomers to firms in skills they have learned; work on publicity and marketing projects where knowledge of a company is a bonus; and in many other ways which would not interfere with the career prospects of the young. Such work is often undertaken on a voluntary basis but if, instead, some of the taxes we pay throughout our lives were designated to create moderate payments for this kind of employment the horror of compulsory retirement from any kind of work would be banished, there would be dignity in continuing to earn a living, and benefits or pensions paid to support those who would rather work, would be cut. A bold and courageous government just might be able to get across the idea that ultimately this may be both more humane and more cost-effective than junking us at the end of mid-life.

There are plenty of consciousness-raising initiatives around this issue, and these should be supported for the sake of future generations as much as for our own. For, shortly after the bulge-and-boom times in which today's mid-lifers were born, the birthrate began to fall. The drop in birthrate since the 1970s means there is a shortage of young people to go into the workplace – a fall which has meant a 25 per cent decline between 1986 and 1995 and similar shortfalls are experienced throughout Europe while in America statistics show that there will be 5 million fewer eighteen- to twenty-four-year-olds in 1995 than there are today, yet the economy in that period is expected to generate 16 million new jobs, many of them requiring a considerable level of education or technical training. There are signs that employers are beginning to realize that they need older employees, as will be discussed, but that is not enough. It is up to us, at mid-life, to use the thrusting, me-first abilities of the 1980s to assert ourselves and insist that we are not just employed but valued for what we are, and that we are described for what we are, rather than what we are not.

But we are not there yet and the truth is that many of us may be offered work on a negative ticket. That may not be particularly cheering but it is better than nothing and something we should turn to our advantage. It is often necessary to use a situation such as this to make points and change public attitudes. It would be nice to think that when, in the 1980s the Prime Minister criticized fixed-age retirement as 'anachronistic', it was in recognition of the value of older workers for what they are. But political cynicism is too well known for us to believe the interest now being shown in mature employees is a road to Damascus conversion.

There is, too, another aspect to this situation. Tom Schuller and Alan Walker point out that, as well as doing all we can to help those who wish to work, we need to protect those who wish to retire at the age promised, but who, because their skills are in limited supply, may be pressurized into staying on at work. They note wryly that: 'The Government's dramatic change of heart reflects the twin pressures of demographic change, leading to an ageing workforce, and directives on equal treatment from the EC.'

Lucy McIntyre laughs when she hears this: 'I applied for a job as a clerk with a small company in the north of England. I was absolutely charmed because they were so enthusiastic about me and I thought they had only read my reference which was very good and hadn't seen my age because I'd assumed they would lose interest then. But they clearly knew that because the woman interviewing me filled in my date of birth of a form. I gathered later from a colleague that, until about two years ago there was an absolute no-no on anyone over thirty being employed but that it had got progressively harder for them to find suitable younger people.'

Dan Ball experienced something similar: 'I applied for a job in a department store and I actually said – gauche I suppose – at the interview that I hoped at forty-four I wasn't too old. The man interviewing just said, "Not at all. You appear very competent and to know what we want." I felt immensely chuffed but I have friends who have had completely the opposite experience.'

There are other small but significant signs that things are shifting and one is the growth of recruitment agencies for the fifties-plus. Jeffrey Ellison, describing his company Age Works, noted: 'There is a realization that older workers need less training, stay longer and because they have experience to draw on, have more to give.' A realization that Ken Dychtwald, director of Age Wave Inc. in California, has also seen, and he is optimistic about the way things will be, envisioning a great need for the experience and training older people have. Once again, in Dychtwald's book, we are seen as generations who will be given the opportunity to break some of the taboos on age, and at the same time demonstrate that today's mid-life and ageing population has a great deal to offer.

It may be that full-time work at the pitch expected of younger people may not be the best or happiest solution for everyone. Part-time and flexible work need to be looked into as a way which might benefit everyone, easing up the pressure on maturing employees, giving time for them to develop other interests and to re-structure their lives before they do eventually retire. Indeed organizational psychologist Professor Carey Cooper at Manchester University, who monitored 1200 early retirees aged fifty to fifty-nine, found that these people did not suffer loss of identity and trauma, but many went into less stressful part-time work and found it very fulfilling. On the other hand those who feel their only hope is to keep on in full-time work, driven by the fear of being seen not to match the youngsters and hoping to climb still higher, can suffer a good deal. He says: 'There are people who have unrealistic goals and think they will make it to the top. They can become very negative.'

One of the schemes which has proved popular in America is flexible retirement which allows people to work out when they might like to retire rather than being presented with an immutable final date before they feel ready to go, and the great virtue of this idea is that it does away with ageism because there is no longer a set time when people are suddenly too old to work. Tom Schuller and Alan Walker spell out in detail their ideas for flexible retirement in *The Time of Our Life* and, along with other campaigning organizations, suggest that flexible retirement should be on offer between the ages of sixty and seventy for men and women with a partial retirement scheme built in to allow for part-time work.

But retirement as we know it is what many of us may well experience, for all the new approaches which are being tried. It will be the sudden shock of going to work one day and having no place there the next. There is something quite chilling about the idea of the goodbye ceremony and then shapeless time stretching ahead. When this happens, whether earlier or later, because of sudden redundancy or the statutary end to a working life, the question that needs asking is how can we avoid the dreadful sense of pointlessness and uselessness so often experienced?

Lilian Ffoulkes, who runs FOCUS pre-retirement courses for businesses, believes it essential that people who are reluctantly leaving work have an opportunity to discuss the things which worry them in individual counselling if they wish, and to draw up plans for re-structuring life afterwards. There are ways this process may be made positive and constructive she says, citing people who have been genuinely enthusiastic about a retirement they were dreading earlier, adds Ffoulkes. She lists the things she covers usually with groups of people within a company which employs her to run the courses. These include the possibility of re-training, education or volunteer work and the need to look at money management. She says: 'It is too easy for people who feel traumatized at what is happening to think there is no point, or to not want to think about it. But as with most things once you confront the situation and become positive and pro-active about it, it is possible to be constructive. I have been delighted at seeing how many of the people who come to the courses really do see that the next bit of life just may be an adventure not a disaster.'

Planning for retirement is big business in America where companies have acknowledged it can make a considerable difference to how their employees cope and, apart from being humanitarian, they have also realized it pays dividends. Ill health and absenteeism have been found to be less in companies where these initiatives are organized. Pre-retirement seminars include a range of things from newsletters, health and welfare support, direct care assistance, social activities which are still open to employees after leaving the company. Counselling and guidance 'lifespan future planning' is widespread and is often offered as far in advance as the beginning of the fifties. But few British companies offer it at present and an EC seminar on Preparation for Retirement found that only 5–10 per cent of those retiring receive any formal help. Charles Handy, Patron of the Re-Action Trust and author of two books on work and retirement, *The Age of Unreason* and *The Empty Raincoat*, suggests pre-retirement care may make the difference between us feeling despair and a sense of control over the future.

Those who retire with skills which have a marketplace value may, of course, end up with the best of all worlds. Columnist Keith Waterhouse paints a cheering scenario: 'Retirement . . . is no longer a matter of wandering – or rather, after all that boardroom sherry, staggering – into the sunset with a mantelpiece clock or barometer under your arm and devoting your days to golf and gardening. Consultancy is the name of the game. You clear your desk on Friday and on Monday – or after that winter cruise – you are re-hired as a freelance consultant. Firms with the nous to buy in expertise are waking up to it at last that the over-fifties have know-how in abundance. They have forgotten things the whiz-kids have yet to learn.' While Ken Dychtwald talks of teams of skilled on-call individuals, people who are invited in for particular projects and others who provide a kind of roving think tank.

Marketing our skills in a way which does not mean a company must offer us full-time employment, is clearly good sense, and mid-lifers who have grown up in entrepreneurial times are well placed to consider how they could best carve a niche for themselves this way. Martin Haig, now in his late fifties, worked in public relations for two decades. When his company went bust during the recession he says: 'I panicked but luckily I have a wonderfully unflappable wife who told me to calm down, see that even if the company didn't still exist, I did, and my abilities were still there. I designed a kind of curriculum vitae and added a couple of sample descriptions of how I approached different commissions, a piece about my philosophy and a final strong statement about why I thought I would be worth their while employing to design projects. I sent it out to hundreds of companies and out of that came a lot of work. In fact I'm as busy as I was but I have a good deal more freedom than I had before.'

Annette Jack was retired from her teaching job and went into despair and felt she was outside the real world. She says: 'I was in mourning and just saw that things had ended for me. My marriage has long been gone, my kids have left home, and I could see nothing but emptiness. Then a friend, older than I am, gave me a very sharp lecture and pointed out that there are plenty of people wanting tutoring. I hadn't thought of that but I put my name down with an agency and put the word around through friends. Within a month I had two pupils, and now, a year later, I work fifteen hours a week which is thoroughly enjoyable and keeps me solvent. I've started taking a course in ancient Greek, something I always wished I'd learnt and which I just might go on to teach afterwards. Then I have time to have lunch with friends. Life has worked out well.'

Jack Mead was made redundant from the plumbers where he had worked for twenty years along with 'a good mate'. They set up in business as freelances which involved no more cost than buying a van, a few extra tools and a spare telephone line in a small room at Jack's home which they use as an office. Jack laughs thinking of the card they had designed: 'We decided to go for humour and had this real toff trying to stem the flow in his pipe with a bandage while water flooded all over the smart furniture. And then we just put, "Let us plumb the depths for you." It worked a treat. We got lots of work quite quickly and although there are lean times when everybody's plumbing seems to behave itself, we both feel, three years on, that we were right to go it alone.'

It seems quite appropriate that those of us who have had the advantages of the best of the post-war opportunities should have to use our inventiveness when things are not going our way. But that possibility does not exist for those people – they are increasing in number and are likely to continue doing so – who find themselves having to care, full time, for a disabled partner or relative. It is something an increasing number of mid-lifers who form a substantial part of the current 6.8 million carers – largely women – in Britain and Europe, are realizing very well. It is a role some have taken on because they do not wish their partners or relatives to go into a home, but others have had the job thrust upon them by the fact that there are not enough residential places, unless they can afford the substantial cost of them. In Britain the Care in the Community legislation, trumpeted by the government as a civilized way forward has, in fact, forced many mid-lifers with ageing parents or relatives to take on full-time responsibility. The government funding for caring for the elderly and infirm is so low that it usually covers just the very minimum of help.

So, at a time when those in the middle years are feeling particularly vulnerable about how they will cope, they are being forced to give up careers and jobs they will not easily get into again, in order to devote their time to caring.

Not surprisingly there is a high level of stress. Jill Pittkeithley, director of the National Carers' Association, points out that some 65 per cent of carers report that their own physical or mental health has been adversely affected by this 'informal' job.

Lucianne Sawyer is a vigorous and outspoken woman whose personal circumstances turned her into an active campaigner. She had taken aged and infirm parents to live in her home because she did not want them to go into a home. She was a single parent with two children and became increasingly worn down by the relentlessness of her days' work and the feeling of trying, entirely on her own, to deal with disability she was in no way qualified to handle. She describes: 'Both my parents were incontinent. My father was wandering around in a confused state leaving his shoes on the table or putting them in the fridge, constantly taking his clothes off. My mother had Alzheimer's disease and even though I had every meal with them and I tried to have coffee and tea with them as well, I would frequently come downstairs and ten minutes later find my mother at the top of the stairs screaming because she had forgotten I had just been up and she thought she was alone in the house.'

Lucianne's personal experience confirmed what she had found while doing government research into why care at home for 500 elderly people had broken down – because there was no respite for them. It was this that inspired her to set up Care Alternatives, an organization providing user-friendly, flexible and appropriate respite care at prices which could be afforded by those who cannot manage the high cost of usual private care.

This issue, which very directly affects those at mid-life who frequently have ailing parents, has brought mid-lifers into the political arena and because they are skilled and energetic in their efforts there are signs that they are making an impact. Caring Costs is an umbrella organization bringing together forty-two voluntary organizations to fight a test case in the European court which won the not particularly generous but nevertheless vital Invalid Care Allowance for married women. Ken Kelling at Caring Costs believes it essential that those who see the need get noisy about it and campaign for improvements that are badly needed. He foresees the possibility of a real crisis if circumstances for carers are not improved. He says: 'We'll have a growing population of frail elderlies and it may be that people will simply not want to care for them because the price is too high. We want to see the state provide a benefit which recognizes the fact that you might have had to give up paid work to care or that it might be difficult to get a job because you are a carer.'

There is a double bind in this situation. On the one hand the lack of resources given to caring for the disabled elderly is one more reflection of ageism which means they are marginalized. On the other side, the fact that women are far and away the largest number of carers, in a society which still sees women as being the ones who are there to nurture and look after the family, means an unspoken assumption that they should be devoting themselves to caring. Would it be the same, I wonder, if men were giving up their careers in equal numbers? Yet poverty is a very real problem amongst older women who for various reasons – bringing up children, caring for aged parents, because after a long marriage in which they devoted themselves to supporting a partner they are left with very little – have few resources to draw on as they age.

The matters I have covered here may not be a direct product of ageism, but it is easy to see how the attitude that older people matter less than younger people, that they have less to offer and can therefore be done unto in a way that suits policy-makers but that has little to do with humanity, has a lot to do with ageism. When we consider a group of people to have less worth than others, then discrimination and lack of compassion somehow become sanctioned. Tom Schuller and Alan Walker predict that ageism will emerge as an issue attracting public and political attention in the 1990s in the same way that sexism and racism emerged as issues in previous decades.

And if anyone can do it, it may well be us. We have had a very different experience from a parent generation which learned the virtue of stoicism, of putting up and shutting up. Today's middle-ager is used to setting agendas, has been involved with women's rights and racial equality, and, as Vic Seidler, forty-six, recalls, the raison d'être of left-wing activists like himself has been the fight against social injustice. He has no doubt that if the rights of old people are not to deteriorate further causing suffering to those already in the firing line, and perhaps establishing a status quo where the elderly who must rely on state benefit will suffer the most diminishing poverty, it is the generations used to flexing their muscles and with a strong sense of their own entitlement, who must get moving.

And it is right that we should all be involved in the battle against ageism. We all age and so are all vulnerable and amongst those who offered me their thoughts for this book there was, over and over again, anger and unhappiness at what getting old may mean in our society. Not everyone does suffer by any means – indeed there is research demonstrating a high level of contentment among some older people – but the point is that enough people do, partly, at least, because of society's way of viewing those who are no longer young. Getting people of all ages, class and circumstances, as well as policy-makers and organizations, to start thinking about ageing is the aim of the charity Age Concern with its Coming of Age campaign which emphasizes that 'tomorrow's older people will be more than statistics, they will be individuals. People like you and me'.

We need to add our weight to organizations like the Grey Panthers, the Associations of Retired Persons here and in

America, and the vigorous trade unionist Jack Jones who leads the UK's Pensioners' Party, helping them fight on behalf of themselves. The importance of older people using political clout is stressed by Gilly Crosbie at the Centre for Policy on Ageing, who expresses frustration that 'older people don't use their vote. There has been a lot of talk about the untapped resource'. If we can join with them and persuade them to do so we will be helping to drive a political initiative that will benefit us when we pass from mid-life into the next life stage. Crosbie, contemplating the growing percentage of the population which is ageing, believes: 'If older people used their vote they would have fantastic power, they could really get listened to and get things changed.'

It is a particularly unpleasant effect of ageism, that older people have been made to feel sufficiently unimportant that they do not fight for their rights but allow themselves to be done unto. That is surely not how we want it to be for our future and if we are to avoid it we need to start thinking about what we will do. As UN Secretary, General Boutros Ghali, suggested the first step is to re-frame an ageing society as a challenge not a burden and when in 1991 the UN General Assembly adopted a set of Principles for Older Persons based on what seems right now, a Utopian Declaration on the Rights and Responsibilities of Older Persons, he urged that young and old and those in-between set themselves the task of re-defining what ageing means. To do this we must start with ourselves and our own attitudes and we would do well to listen to the point he made: 'It will require a new view of themselves by those who are ageing and a new view on the part of . . . those who have not yet aged.'

That will do as a ground plan but shouldn't we go further than that, bearing in mind the success of the Grey Panthers in getting themselves seen, heard and acknowledged, do as Maggie Kuhn has done, and think outrageous?

To understand just why ageism has reached the degree of unpleasantness described at the beginning of this chapter we need to understand the implications of demographic changes.

It is in the workplace – or all too often out of it – that the middle-aged first become most acutely aware of age as a handicap. With this realization the demographic 'time-bomb' – another threatening, war-related metaphor to describe the new generations of elders – has become a political issue. But not, as might seem appropriate, bringing political focus on how best to care for the increased number of old people, and what sort of structures and system could be set up to care for future generations. The situation may not be as extreme for today's thirty-year-olds for example, when they reach retirement age, but nor is it likely to be as well protected for them as it has been in the past. Those who have already reached middle age and realize how tough things ahead may be are viewing the future with anxiety. A survey of older people throughout Europe for the European Year of Older People (1993) found 'quite a high level of pessimism and uncertainty about whether or not the state would continue to take care of older people' and less than one in three felt confident enough in the future of their country's Welfare State to believe it would look after them. Gordon Marriott, in his late fifties, approaches older age with 'a certain amount of trepidation' and says that he does not see much positive about the ageing process because: 'The social and economic system in the UK is against that.' The fear of poverty is uncomfortably real even though he worked until he was made redundant in his fifties and paid towards the pension he believed the government would give him to ensure a level of security in later life.

We need a climate where it is seen as politically disgraceful if resourcing for their needs is cut. Schuller and Walker see a covert and damaging ageism in the way older people are categorized as needy or particularly needy, deserving or less deserving of resources. They see it as vital that personal and social attitudes to older people 'come under increasing scrutiny, calling into question the assumptions which underlie public policy and individual behaviours ... the way in which the boundary is drawn between those who are old and those who are not is, to some extent at least, a matter of social and economic policy. This affects, in ways which are still very dimly understood, the views that older people have of themselves.'

Why, one wonders, have they put up with it so passively? The answer lies surely in the fact that they are generations accustomed to having little power and who will usually accept what is done to them. For many of today's elders, who have been through two world wars, putting up and shutting up is what they assume must be done. That feeling needs to be translated into action and there are signs that this is happening to some degree. An increasing number of individuals and organizations working on behalf of older people, believe governments can and should be made to listen, and that ageism must be made the political issue of the 1990s.

Nobody is pretending the situation is easy. The future, in which we seem likely to live longer, is an unknown quantity. Today's obituaries exclaiming at the impressive lifespan of ninety-year-olds and even the Queen's 100th birthday telegram may become commonplace. Policy-makers cannot be sure for what sort of numbers, over what sort of period and with what level of dependence they must make provision. The words from the Re-Action Trust, a joint initiative between British Industry and Help the Aged which aims to change corporate policy towards the retired and elderly recognizes this: 'If we are to avoid major social and economic problems, the implications of the dramatic rise of the Third Age will require a radical reappraisal by businesses and government as well as individuals.' While the authors of the major Eurobarometer survey which looked at experiences and attitudes of older people throughout Europe talked of 'an enormous challenge' to governments and to everyone involved in economic and social life. In grim terms John Ermisch at the National Institute for Economic and Social Research in his report *Fewer Babies, Longer Lives* observed: 'Intergenerational political strife over whether pensions of the children of the 1960s should be cut, or greater burdens placed on a smaller workforce, seems certain and needs to be thought about now.'

Ermisch is right and what is needed is a radical look at how social protection, employment policies, health policies and housing policies can be structured and financed. Perhaps they cannot remain precisely as they are now but what we have seen in Britain is a crude and peculiarly unkind type of political sleight of hand effectively reducing the benefits and care which have been the right of fourth-agers since Beveridge's welfare state came into being. In the 1980s the Conservative Government's modified SERPS (State Earnings-related Pensions Scheme) the national insurance policy for the elderly, for which most have trustingly paid throughout their working lives believing they would be provided for in older age. Alongside this were changes in housing benefits so that pensioners lost certain entitlements, and in the 1990s the Tories brought in the Community Care Act which has the sound principle of keeping elderly people in their homes and communities, but has been so under-resourced that many have had to rely on family and relatives to give up jobs and act as full-time carers. Others have simply suffered in the way of Daisy who is past retirement age, has bad arthritis and lives alone in a flat. She cannot get out of bed by herself let alone go down the stairs and into the streets. The council has funded twice-a-day care – she is visited some time between 8 a.m. and midday and got out of bed, put into a chair and left. A neighbour pops in most days and puts a tin of soup into the microwave, stops for a chat then goes. Daisy's evening care call to put her to bed is between 5 pm and 9 pm. She says: 'I just sit most of the day and watch the TV. If I'm feeling very restless I try to hobble around the flat but that's not much fun and I fell one time. Sometimes the carer stays and has a cup of tea with me but she's often in a hurry. If I had the money I'd pay someone to keep me company a bit. I miss the feeling of someone around and I like conversation, but I can't do that on my pension so I just have to get on with life as it is.'

Standing charges for amenities such as water were introduced – a new expenditure for pensioners and VAT was put on to the price of fuel. One way and another things have got progressively worse for older people while politicians warn that things may never be as good as they have been again. And this at a time when, reports Social Europe, three-quarters of EC respondents think their governments do not do enough for older people and there is considerable poverty, although this is somewhat less in countries where they have relatively progressive policies on the elderly such as Denmark, the Netherlands, Luxembourg and France.

The genesis of the dismissive ageism we see today is depicted with cringe-making accuracy in William Trevor's short story 'Broken Homes' where a teacher from a local comprehensive is 'persuading' eighty-seven-year-old Mrs Malby into allowing a group of his pupils from broken homes in to decorate her kitchen 'as an experiment in community relations'. Mrs Malby's obvious anxiety, her explaining that she did not want the kitchen re-decorated, her request to be left as she is, are pushed aside in the way the words of a none-too-bright toddler's might be, as the teacher tells her he thinks her a 'love' and 'absolutely splendid for eighty-seven' and, over-riding her objections, has her home decorated in a manner and colour which leave her in abject misery. For all that, cowed by anxieties about how the state could deal with her if she became troublesome, Mrs Malby says nothing.

Such attitudes did not diminish through the years, but the belief that older people deserve to be cared for did. Annabel Brodie-Smith, at the University of Syracuse, describes this in her article 'A "Grey" Area', and sees, expediently, a damaging latter-day image of elders as feisty and up-and-at-'em which has presumably been selectively drawn from the politically motivated Grey Panthers and relatively well-off active 'golden oldies', as they are tagged. But in the US as well as in Europe these images, which legitimize the 'pension snatcher' kind of hostility, are only part of a picture which is dominated at least as much by the increasingly embattled and defeated-feeling elders who see their welfare as a low priority. Brodie-Smith explains: 'In the 1960s and early 1970s, elderly people were portrayed as poor and deserving and therefore universal, benevolent policies were implemented to assist them. However, during the 1980s the image of the elderly changed to the equally misleading perception of them as vibrant, powerful and financially secure and whose costly government programmes were bursting the federal budget in the USA.'

In Europe more than 70 per cent of people now live to seventy years and the numbers are increasing. Just a century ago the number achieving this age was only 20 per cent. It is this change which has brought the focus sharply on to workplace ageism and enforced retirement with organizations such as the Carnegie Trust, the Re-Action Trust and the Centre for Policy on Ageing, battling for change and to raise awareness of its importance as a political issue.

Yet all the pre-retirement help in the world cannot dispel the misery caused to people who are forced to live a borderline existence, constantly worried about money, when they retire.

And this is how it is for a great many people throughout Europe who rely on state pensions for the last stage of their lives. There is a familiar pattern, explain the authors of 'Older People in Europe: Social and Economic Policies', which shows that as people cross the third-age threshold of fifty they become progressively less reliant on salaries and wages and more reliant on pensions. This is fine for those who have supplemented what the state will give with private pension schemes, but for those who have not been in a position to do so and who have no other source of income, poverty is a very real problem. The big-brother handout places the state in a special relationship with older people and emphasizes the vital importance of public policy in determining the living standards of this group, explains the authors. It means that in countries such as Denmark and the Netherlands where social responsibility has a high priority they do not debate who is or is not eligible but give a pension to all citizens. But looking after the elderly is given very different priority in different countries. The highest level is 16.9 per cent of the national income which, in 1984, was what Italy allotted, while Britain gave less than half of this and, as Schuller and Walker point out, the government 'has already acted to curtail severely the future growth of pension expenditure'. And projected spending tells blatantly how much worse the British Government is prepared to treat a section of the public which has no fall-back position. By the year 2020 Britain will spend 8.6 per cent of the GDP while the figure is 21.6 per cent for France and 25.6 per cent in Italy.

Pensioners' incomes in the UK have been reduced in relation to average earnings over the last decade, saving £4000 million – a piece of treatment which contrasts starkly with the action of the French government which has sought to raise the incomes of older people by extending the coverage of social assistance and where retirement pensions are indexed to net wages or prices, whichever is higher. A reflection of Italy's relatively generous spending on pensioners is reflected in a growth in living standards over the last 40 years which is higher than the general EC population.

But with the large majority of Europeans over retirement age receiving their income from public pension the issue of widespread hardship is very real. Eurobarometer surveyors asked retirees whether pensions they received, and they included private pensions, were adequate and found a relatively high level of frustration at not being able to lead a desired lifestyle. It would be cheering if people were prepared to put money where their mouths are, to know that in many EC countries the general public believes that the main problem facing older people is not having enough to live on. Ironically in the UK, where fear that pensions may be cut with the demographic changes has been demonstrably real under the Conservative government, the concern is high at 66 per cent of the population, whereas in Denmark, where pensions are being reformed and constructive ways of funding investigated, only a quarter of people believe elders must suffer financially.

To Tom Hoyes, a retired civil servant, who has become extremely active on behalf of the aged, battling to ensure that pensions are safeguarded and provide a realistic support for the elderly in need, is a top priority. Jack Jones, of the Pensioners' Party undoubtedly raised awareness of pensioners' plight with his protests over the government's decision to put VAT on the price of fuel. Hoyes believes: 'We have to go to battle over it, and we need to draw in professionals who know how best to do it. Look at the campaign that won war widows their increase – it was successful because it used public relations, drawing in Harry Secombe and Vera Lynn. We also need pensioners to get noisy about their lot, to stand up publicly at demonstrations and on TV and say here's my pension, here's my electricity bill and water bill, my council tax. You can see I get seventy-five pounds and I pay out eighty pounds so please tell me how I'm supposed to live? The problem is it's not happening. There needs to be more pensioner representation on various bodies to make older people more visible. I'm going to a course on Pensioner Power next week to learn more about how to get noticed.'

Women not only suffer age discrimination but they also suffer greater poverty because of gender. The authors of *Older People in Europe* show that women get markedly lower pensions than men throughout almost the entire EC, and they attribute this to the different treatment of men and women by social policies except in Denmark which has a flat rate for men and women.

The degree of scaremongering which has been generated at the idea of grey generations draining resources because of an excessive need for health care and support, has, as discussed earlier, created a climate where it is possible for government to actually say that it may be too expensive to fund long-term medical care, or to carry out life-or-death operations on the elderly. Apart from the obvious cruelty of instilling in elders the idea that care at a stage in life when ill health can be particularly distressing, can no longer be afforded, this scare-mongering also disguises truths about just how much older people actually use in terms of resources. Annabel Brodie-Smith says angrily that the belief that the elderly are an economic and social burden because of physiological deterioration and environmental constraints is unjustified: 'The image of older people as frail, dependent and diseased is a serious distortion of the true picture. The majority of older people live healthy and happy lives. Only about one in twenty elderly people in the OECD (Organization of Economic Cooperation and Development) countries are resident in a geriatric institution, and in England only one in ten receives visits from any public social service.'

Demonstrating this point are the findings of a survey done in Manchester into 39,000 consultations with GPs which show that the over-seventy-five-year-olds who accounted for 6 per cent of the survey's population, made only 8 per cent of the consultations. And that percentage had decreased in the past ten years. Yet the government's alarmist talk when they published their Green Paper, 'The Health of the Nation', implying that the prevention of illness in adult life would merely postpone it to later life, was an 'uninformed opinion' criticizes Brodie-Smith, and potentially extremely damaging.

The authors of *Age and Attitudes* (Eurobarometer Survey) also had things to say on this matter, finding that across Europe just one-third of those between sixty and sixty-four reported a limiting long-standing illness or disability, and the figure rose to nearly half at aged eighty and over, but even in the eldest age group the majority did not regard themselves as disabled to any major extent. And the significant point, if we are considering the cost of help, is that just 18 per cent of sixty- to sixty-four-year-olds were getting care, although the needs of fourth-agers of eighty years and over were higher, with 59 per cent needing help.

It is also ironic that, while public angst is whipped up over how care of elders will be funded, the vast majority of those who become too ill to cope, requiring full-time care do not get it from the state but from their partners or a member of their family, and it is only in the eighty-plus age groups that the state provides a slightly higher percentage of care, presumably to people whose partners have died or can no longer cope. It has been estimated that some 6 million people providing informal care for someone who is elderly, sick or handicapped save the British taxpayer between £15 and £24 billion a year.

These figures are ammunition with which to fight the propaganda suggesting elders are gobbling up resources with their health needs. They also debunk the myth, as Alan Walker comments, that families are less willing than they were to care for their families.

This may be encouraging at a time when the belief in the breakdown of family, that loving human bonds are ever weakening, has become a kind of conventional wisdom and the degree of commitment shown here, even allowing for those caring unwillingly and with stiff upper lip, tells a very different story. What has been achieved so far may not match the aspirations of the campaigning groups but it is undoubtedly several steps on from passive acceptance. The Association of Directors of Social Services in the UK have come out in favour of rights and entitlements for carers.

Looking back at the issues which so affect elders, how rife and unchallenged the discrimination is against them, and how easily their needs and well-being may be made into the unacceptable face of public expenditure, the importance of making ageing a political issue becomes very clear. It may be that midlifers are the ones who must use their expertise at being activists to set the agenda, but it is also important that elders themselves stand up and are heard and counted.

Looking Forward

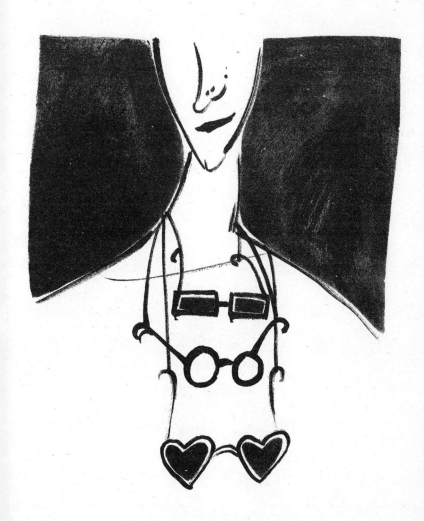

> What better way . . . to celebrate a seventieth year
> than with a feast of friends? And if I had imagined this year as one
> with time for reflection, it is always a mistake to try to order one's
> life in such an arbitrary way . . . Right now just three days' rest and
> holiday are all that I need to reset my course, as happy and
> free as a sailor putting out again into the ocean
> after anchoring in a sheltered bay.
>
> MAY SARTON, *On Being Seventy*

H E STORMED ON TO the stage with a hop, a skip and a
mighty swagger. His voice was a megaphone of enthusiasm one minute, a hefty berating tone the next broken often
with a howl of 'Shut Up!' sending us, the almost entirely
middle-aged audience packing out the Wembley Arena, into
paroxysms of delight and laughter. Then, suddenly he was
sitting at the piano pounding out those songs we remembered
so well: 'Shake, Rattle and Roll', 'My Blue Heaven', 'Good
Golly Miss Molly', and many, many more. Here was Little
Richard back on stage in Britain after countless years, 'sixty-
two years young' – as he declared time and again – giving a
billion-octane performance which lasted over two hours and
would have had armies of younger men flat on their backs.
Not Little Richard – his body exercised to the elasticity of an
electric eel, his zest for life firing every cylinder. He gyrated,
jived and jigged until his finale.

What a triumph for age, what a life-enhancing revelation
for the thousands of us contemplating the years ahead, who
had bought tickets for a sentimental journey and found ourselves compelled to dance in the aisles, to clap and shout as the
notes which seemed to hurl themselves from the piano, awak-
ened the youngsters we had been when we heard them first
time around. For an evening we were caught up in a euphoria
which rendered us ageless and unageing in our minds and
bodies. But like Cinderella returning to her life as scullery
maid, we must understand that such transformations are time

out of time, that Little Richard is a grand exception to the rules about ageing. Mustn't we?

The short answer is no we must not, and should not, unless we actually want to take part in the over-practised business of self-fulfilling prophecy, and my aim here is to present the evidence for looking forward with optimism and enthusiasm.

The number of mid-lifers growing into old age is, as we have seen, rising steadily. It is estimated in *Social Europe*, the publication based on research done during the International Year of Older People and Solidarity Between Generations, that Europe's population of over-sixties (68.6 million in 1993) will have doubled by 2020. Five years later, in 2025 Americans over sixty-five are set to outnumber teenagers by more than two to one, it is projected that by the year 2050 one-fifth of the world's projected population – 2.5 billion people – will be sixty-five or older. In earlier chapters I have looked at the problems which may arise around mid-life and which are connected to the business of ageing, the issues we need to address sooner rather than later if old age is to be the best not the worst we can achieve. I have homed in on the drawbacks to being the demographic bulge generations. But in this chapter I intend to focus on what may be positive about time ahead.

This is a unique time for the ageing population and there are many reasons why there is virtue in numbers. The ongoing efforts of researchers and scientists to endlessly improve the prognosis for our bodies, the efforts of designers, entrepreneurs, manufacturers to meet our needs with an alacrity not known before are direct results of our people power. As it sinks in that we have a substantial chunk of the West's disposable income in our piggy banks, so we see all kinds of organizations, services, enterprises coming to being, in order to provide for us, and there can be little doubt that all this will impact on and alter for the better how we are viewed and treated as we get older. It is a point Neil Mackwood made, writing in the *Sunday Times*, identifying what he sees as a significant shift in the *Zeitgeist*: 'There is an emotional sea-change going on. It is as though we are on the cusp of growing up.'

That is encouraging, not least because it should mean that older people, their lives, activities, ideas and philosophies will become a subject of interest and if that happens we might listen to what the voices from the front have to say. Rather than simply being prone to the negative messages, convinced by the fashionable blanking out of older people's lives and experiences, convinced that there can be nothing of value to know, we might set about learning what elders who have crossed the mid-life rubicon and moved into the uncharted territory of later life, feel about the way it is out there. It is well worth doing, as I now know from having researched this chapter, from having found older people who do not see old age as a regret, devoid of meaning because they no longer have what they had when younger. Rather they see themselves as having done their time on the tasks of earlier life – bringing up children, investing their time and energy in making a living, building careers, and that now they are liberated from the constraints these things impose. I talked with, heard from and read about older people full of vigour and enthusiasms, who were and are taking up new challenges, making plans, fulfilling lifelong ambitions and delighting in the fact that there is now time to broaden their minds, improve their bodies, spend time with partners and put more energy than has been possible before into friendships.

This is, of course, a selective picture because it leaves out the saddening and shaming fact that a percentage of older people's lives are blighted by poverty, illness, loneliness and a sense of being disenfranchised – things for them are every bit as bad as the grim pictures we carry of what ageing means and there is no way we should be sanguine about the way these elders' needs are undervalued. But this is something I have looked at in an earlier chapter, and it seems important to recognize that they are not the majority. A great many older people live lives of considerable satisfaction and pleasure in spite of the increasing problems of health and physique which go with ageing; the recognition that our bits will not do what they used to as described wryly by American comedian Bill Cosby in *Time Flies*, his reflection on turning fifty: 'A few days ago a friend tried to cheer me up by saying "Fifty is what forty used to be." He had made an inspirational point: and while I ponder it, my forty-year-old-knees are suggesting I sit down and my forty-year-old eyes are looking for their glasses, whose location has been forgotten by my forty-year-old mind.'

When older people throughout the European states were surveyed it was found that at least two-thirds are active in some way, and another survey measuring levels of satisfaction found that more than half the older people were fairly satisfied with their lives, just under a quarter were very satisfied and just one in five did not feel satisfied. Still more encouraging was the result of a British survey which concluded that 69 per cent of older people enjoy later life as much and in a third of cases, more than they enjoyed younger life. This finding was echoed by research from America which found that although people moving beyond seventy years regretted a drop in activity, they maintained a sense of self-worth and of satisfaction with past and present life. We hear that in Margaret Worthington's reflection: 'When I bought a car at sixty-five I assumed it would be my last – until at eighty-five I bought a new Mini. I like to think I have gone along with a changing world and I know I get the most out of life by keeping up with it.'

It is there too in the robust response the writer Robert Kastenbaum received when introduced to a woman close to her one hundredth birthday. He asked what she made of life and her reply was: 'Can't tell yet! I'm still making my life!' In similar mood octogenarian Sir Lew Grade saw no reason to start summing up his life: 'I'm eighty-four and I'm just starting.' While Sir John Gielgud, asked on his ninetieth birthday what plans he had for slowing down, was having none of that: 'I'd much rather work'.

If we are to look forward and go forward positively it is

vital that we learn to find a different mind-set to that described by psychologist Jere Daniel in *Psychology Today* magazine which he sees as afflicting the new mid-lifers: 'On the cusp of fifty, having come late into maturity, they can suddenly envision themselves becoming obsolete, just as their fathers, mothers, grandparents, uncles and aunts did when they crossed the age sixty-five barrier, the moment society now defines as the borderline between maturity and old age.' But how do we change the mind-set? We can best do it I believe by opening our eyes and ears, and by adopting the attitude suggested (hopefully as he is only in his early fifties) by my partner, that when we have dealt with our mid-life demons and learned to face the future with greater equanimity, we can see ourselves as 'over the hump but not over the hill'. Because being over the hill tends to be seen as losing the capacity to do the things we have enjoyed when young, or which we would have liked to do when young but feel must be lost dreams when we are older. It is important to see that this may be more to do with what is in our heads than an affliction of the limbs or brain.

It is an irresistible conclusion if you dip into Jeremy Baker's wonderful compilation of information on who did what at different ages, *Tolstoy's Bicycle*, so named because Tolstoy learned to ride a bike aged sixty-seven. Among the myriad assembled examples of older citizens kicking underfoot all the assumptions we have about what is and is not possible in later life, Baker tells us that William Gladstone became prime minister for the fourth time at the age of eighty-two; Chairman Mao could still swim nine miles along the Yalu River in sixty minutes at the age of seventy-five and suffragette Sylvia Pankhurst emigrated to Ethiopia at the age of seventy-four. Just a few examples. And then there is the observation of the musician Pablo Casals, aged ninety-six: 'Age is a relative matter. If you continue to work and absorb the beauty of the world about you, you find that age does not necessarily mean getting old. At least not in the ordinary sense.'

It is indeed relative. I feel a mere stripling contemplating these people and there seems a kind of idiocy in bemoaning my aged state, whereas when I read of the latest appointments to high places, in my profession – or indeed in almost any profession – and realize they are well and truly my juniors, then I feel old. When I learn that, yet again, newspaper supplements and magazines are struggling to appeal to a younger market and to hell with us matured folk who happen to believe we are still people worth communicating with, I feel hurt and upset. It makes me downright angry when I realize that almost all popular entertainment excludes the likes of me, presumably because I'm past my entertaining date. Then there is the constant drip drip of jokes, remarks and ways of addressing anyone over about forty, that are frankly diminishing. It is then that I have a sense of futility about the years ahead and what will be possible.

Perspective is all.

That being the case I decided, as I believe we all must do as part of the challenge of mid-life, to focus on all the evidence there is for the value in age. I found myself visualizing a dinner party of elders whose company would guarantee a vigorous, entertaining and intellectually stimulating evening – the kind of evening youngsters could not match because they lack the *savoir faire*, an evening at which they would not be missed because no way could they be better company. There would be Baroness Barbara Castle, Lord Healey, Edward Heath, from the politicians' pack, writers Ruth Prawer Jhabvala, Gore Vidal and Fay Weldon, gallery owner Angela Flowers whose seasoned sexiness and roguish humour guarantees that any dinner with her is hilarious. Benjamin Spock would get an invite, because he is a continuing explorer of life; Lord Young of Dartington who has tackled most of Britain's social ills in his extensive life, and Nelson Mandela would be a must. Across the table from them would be landscape architect Sir Geoffrey Jellicoe, now in his nineties, film stars Walter Matthau and Sophia Loren, playwright Arthur Miller and Alistair Cooke with his exquisitely compassionate yet unsentimental view of the world. Sir Laurens Van der Post, frail now but still so vigorous in mind and Cristina Hoyos, Spanish prima ballerina of flamenco who performed for the opening ceremony of the Olympic Games with its expectant audience of billions. The list could go on and on.

Indeed the list does go on and on if we include the less well known and those whose activities might not command public attention, but are nevertheless an impressive demonstration of creative, mentally rigorous and physically adventurous lives being lived. Take Margaret and Maureen, both in their late seventies, whose lives are spent travelling the globe; I found my own life as mother of two teenagers and a busy freelance journalist, seeming rather bland and staid by comparison.

Both women were in their fifties when they lost their husbands and, working together, they formed a close supportive friendship. They moved together into a little house in Wembley on the outskirts of London. Both had always wanted to travel and with a great guffaw of laughter Margaret points to the copies of the *National Geographic* magazine which line their sitting room: 'That's what we've done; we've seen a good many of the places in those magazines. It's been terribly interesting, dreadfully exciting at times, and once in a while you're off somewhere and you wish you hadn't gone around the corner! But more often we're just thrilled by what we discover.'

Over the past fifteen years on money saved from their widows' pensions and the odd jobs they do for others, they have visited Russia nine times, been to Belize, the Galapagos islands and South America, where they went whaling. Maureen recalls: 'We went to Mongolia and Siberia and to Australia to see people we had met on our travels.' They tend to start off on package trips because they find it the cheapest way then go off exploring on their own once they have arrived. There have, on occasions, been problems over their age. Margaret says, positively spitting out the words: 'Once or twice I've been asked how old we are when investigating holidays on the phone, and then I'm told we wouldn't be able to keep up, that we'd hinder the others. Oh yes? I say and tell them about the time we went down the Amazon in a canoe, tramped through the rainforest in wellies, climbed the banks and walked through great boulders, while some of the younger members of the party wouldn't do it and couldn't keep up.'

Lou Miller, a one-time Midlands racing cyclist, made a comeback after an absence of thirty years and now he is Events co-ordinator for the Cumbria Section of the League of Veteran Cyclists, an organization brought to life by the frustration of men and some women who wanted to take up cycling in later life and found that established cycling organizations could not offer them the quantity or quality of activities they wanted. These days he organizes events designed, Miller says, to 'challenge the concept that athletic achievement is solely the domain of young people' – rather the opposite as during school holidays fourteen- to sixteen-year-olds join the Veterans and learn from them, while Miller is delighted because, 'Our competitive age-banded events have attracted many former racing cyclists back into the sport and they now line up against rivals they have not seen for thirty years or more.'

There are people who say loudly and clearly how thoroughly they are enjoying the stage of life they are at. Ethel Keane, now in her seventies, is one of many older people whose pleasure in having time to develop her creativity, makes the later years in her view 'the best I have had'. Her earlier life was hard and busy. Widowed young with a child she struggled to make ends meet and bring him up well.

It is in the years since he left home and established a successful life, that she has been able to turn time and attention to developing her painting which has become a passion, an involvement and the focus in a life she speaks of with enviable happiness. She says, 'I started with painting classes locally, I went once a week – most of the others were older people – and I found I could do it, and that it delighted me. I have never minded making a bosh of a picture, the pleasure is in trying to capture something. I feel absolutely elated if I drive down by the river, or along the coastline where I live and see a lovely scene. I just stop and get my easel and paints out and have a go.

'Over the years I have improved and my confidence has grown as I've become more and more able to get the pictures to work as I want, and in the past few years I've had exhibitions and I sell most of my pictures. Sometimes I refuse because I can't bear to part with one I love particularly. The painting takes up most of my time and fills my life.'

I have heard people say there is no point in studying in later life because where does it lead you, but the increasing numbers of retired people studying for degrees, attending courses at the University of the Third Age and local education classes who are developing their knowledge, stretching their intellectual powers in all kinds of other ways, clearly do not share this view.

These are people led by a conviction that there is not a cut-off age for what you can do, rather it is up to us. At Age Resource, the 'younger arm' of Age Concern in England, set up to guide, support and give awards to older people who are becoming 'social entrepreneurs' taking up adventurous pur-suits, volunteering for important work, developing skills and learning and acting as mentors to youngers they explain: 'We don't say "I can't do it because of my age", we say: "I can do it at my age." Just that change of emphasis is important.' Joyce Ridgeway who took up belly-dancing at the age of seventy certainly agrees. When a friend lent her a video of belly-dancing she decided to 'have a go' and she set about making up her own choreography. She was asked by Age Resource to dance at an event with an audience of 2500 people, since which time she has performed regularly in her green chiffon outfit with gold trimmings. It has shaped her life: 'I work with the elderly showing them they don't have to live within four walls. I run a tea dance every week and I've been asked by my peers to run a belly-dancing class.'

Wonderful and inspiring stuff isn't it? Or do we really think it all rather inappropriate? Do we genuinely applaud older people who are saying through their actions, that so long as mind and body are fit there is no reason why they should not do anything a younger person does? Or do we find it quaint and slightly embarrassing, and determine from our mid-life vantage point that we would sooner fade out discreetly, no matter how depressing the prospect may be? Would we be inclined to say, as the television cameraman filming Joyce did: 'Don't you think you are too old to be doing this?'

These are questions we do well to ask ourselves and answer honestly, for how we respond will shape how we go forward. If deep inside we see people like Joyce and Lou as acting inappropriately; if we think that people like Ethel taking up creative tasks as not doing something serious but merely filling the years until death, then we need to acknowledge these feelings. We may hear that overworn cliché, 'You're as young as you feel', slipping off our tongues, knowing there is little conviction to it. The way we react to what may still seem a far-off stage, and to the burgeoning number of older people, fitter and more full of conviction than has usually been true in the past, is, after all, determining the way we will be judging what is possible in our own future.

The reaction of Mo Harter, a single mother approaching her fifties with four almost grown-up children, was enthusiastic when she read what I have written so far: 'It makes me want to get there. When I think of all the things I'd like to do I need years and years and there's no reason why I can't do them as an older and even an old woman provided I stay in one piece. I see the time when my children are gone as time for me and that feels exciting.' But then she hesitated and added: 'If I'm honest I don't feel ready to go into that next stage yet, and I wonder what it takes to make you ready.'

Bob Chambers, now in his mid-fifties, wonders much the same: 'I have an uncle who is the most marvellously spirited chap. He runs a little business he started after retirement and he's always off sailing or windsurfing. He's kept his body in marvellous nick and he's not short of partners if he wants them. In many ways he's got as much as a younger man and he *is* a good role model for later life. Yet I worry about how to get to his stage with the kind of conviction he has.'

These are key questions, the thoughts so many of us have as we travel across the bridge having left the youth camp, and en route to join the elders. During this time we may feel ourselves caught in that state which T. S. Eliot captures so perfectly:

> Time present and time past
> Are both perhaps present in time future
> And time future contained in time past

And we may find we are recognizing that our task is to find a way to bring our two worlds together. Not only that, but to do it in a way that does not mean we are forever hankering for the time which has gone, so that we can carry what we have learned and gained in that part of our existence forward, to enrich the future. Actress Jeanne Moreau talks of having come to that: 'I have a very juvenile feeling of change and a new life. Nothing starts at one specific moment. The older you get the more you realize everything is the fruit of what you are.'

It was just a couple of years ago that I grasped what had been gained in my growing years and how the confidence and conviction acquired would enable me to deal with my world in a way which would have been impossible a few years ago. Quite suddenly I was aware of feeling old enough to be taken seriously. I see it as connected to the tough struggle I had with my despairing feelings earlier; it seemed that that process had enabled me to slough off the persona which had done me well through younger years, but which no longer fitted. The aware-ness was nothing spectacular, it would not have been a con-spicuous change to the outside world, but I was all at once aware that a change had taken place in the way I deal with people, work, friends and my relationship with my partner. Talking on the phone to commissioning editors I heard myself being assertive about the way I would write my articles. Interviewing people beside whom earlier I would have felt lesser and thus intimidated, I found myself talking to them as equals and as a result getting much better interviews; I stopped being acquiescent about behaviour I do not like from my partner and at the same time being more able to see it as reasonable that he may also dislike some of my behaviour. I see all these as the product of a confidence which has come because of years lived, because of what I have experienced, what I know, and also because at this stage in life I am no longer in the middle of the years spent trying to build a career, being careful, employing strategies, fearing incurring displeasure, being so easily shot down by criticism. I have survived this far, and I am as good and as bad as the sum total of the experience. To my surprise I have stopped feeling competitive in the frantic way I used to, a condition my profession inspires – and it is a relief not to be wanting to do again the kind of work I see the generations behind me doing. Rather there is a curiosity and anticipation about what I can, quite quietly, do next. If I can look at what I would like the future to be and see myself as a student of the next stage, looking to the elders I admire as examples and mentors, then there's bags of potential and what I make of that will be very much the product of the things I have learned, the life-skills I have acquired thus far.

Jenny Waters has reached her fifties and sees that the process of living has broadened and matured her in a way that she values. She says: 'My views have moderated considerably as I have got older – a measure of acquired wisdom and tolerance has made me less extreme and I see this as a virtue. However, my ideas have not actually changed – I am still a Labour voter and still believe in all the causes I once supported. The biggest change in terms of values and priorities is that I no longer see work as the most important thing. I was a workaholic for years, which was almost essential in terms of career-building, but now I see work as a means to an end and my priorities focus more on family and friends.'

Cindy Anderson too can see a bargain in her situation. After reflecting on the drawbacks of middle age she says: 'Yet for all this there's a certain poise that comes with middle age too; you've been there, done it, seen the film, eaten the pie, and you know how many beans make five. You can get through the day with some semblance of dignity; you can do your job, run your house, cope with emergencies and problems, and do it all with a quiet smile, while all around you things are happening which in former times would have rendered you homicidal, suicidal, or just plain mean.'

Yet appreciating what we have garnered in our years and being able to see that perhaps it is some kind of preparation for the next stage of growing up, does seem to be harder for men still involved in competitive careers where they may be striving to keep up with younger employees and where their knowledge and experience is overshadowed by the fact that they are older. It is hard too for men who see retirement and being forced out of the role which has moulded their life for so many years, as the end of anything they can imagine making sense of – a situation that has been looked at in an earlier chapter.

There are, however, men who speak as readily as do the women quoted, about the rewards of life lived. Playwright Hugh Whitemore, in his late fifties, talks of the worth of the confidence he has gained, and indeed he seems full of equanimity at the prospect of moving into the next decade. The years he has spent reading, studying subjects as research for his plays – among them *A Pack of Lies* and *Breaking the Code*, both of which played in the West End – and in conversation with other intellectuals, have made him wonderfully informed and entertaining. But the reason he believes older age (other than dying with which he hasn't yet come to terms) seems to offer possibilities and new opportunities is because: 'I live in my head and I am forever learning new things which add to what I already know. With the amassing of knowledge I find myself working out new ideas for plays, stories – whatever. I think if what goes on in your head continues to be exciting then you do not have to dread ageing unless you go dotty. I do feel anxious about my mind going, but there again look at old Shaw: he went dotty and wrote awful things in his nineties thinking they were good, but the point is it probably doesn't matter if you remain convinced.'

For others the value of what has been learned in early years is that it provides a bank from which they can draw in order to change direction. Tony Neate, in his fifties, knew he was taking a risk leaving a career with a multi-national company where he seemed likely to go on progressing, but felt compelled to do so because 'day after day I felt more miserable about going to work'. Had he made the same change of direction, setting up healing and spiritual courses in the country in younger years, he doubts he would have been knowledgeable or skilled enough in the important business basics to succeed. He is in his sixties now, making this point, and explains that he then applied the concentration he has also mastered through the years to learning about healing and spiritualism, so that now he has a new life-style which continues to evolve. He says: 'I feel I have the maturity and knowledge to run the centre as a going concern and I see the years ahead as tremendously exciting because they are an opportunity for me to learn so many things which I can bring to the centre. If I look at my life it seems to have a logic, a continuum.'

If we are convinced our young years have been the time of our life, and that anything later can only be less, then obviously the prospect of getting older may be tough. But the irony is that for all the hype and celebration of youth, the years from teens to mid-life are often marred by the difficult business of learning how to deal with it, how to tackle the complex goals before us. If we cast our minds back and recall, young life probably had as many worries, problems, uncertainties and anxieties as does later life. Plenty of the people who have shared their thoughts on ageing with me, have observed this and even those who find the prospect of losing the opportunities of youth, the look of youth, very hard, insist they do not actually want to BE young again. There is a good deal of sense in Lord Asquith's observation that 'Youth would be an ideal state if it came a little later in life.' And by the time we reach mid-life there's a fair chance of having what Steve talks of as 'the knowledge of survival'. He explains: 'At least now, as a fifty-year-old I know I've got through difficulties, pains, depressions, things which seemed insoluble at the time, and I've come out the other side smiling. That's worth a lot.' Or we may recognize ourselves in Janet: 'I looked at older people whose lives seemed so worked out when I was younger and wondered if and how I could achieve that. The fact I apparently had all this wonderful youth didn't really seem to mean much. I look at my daughter now and I don't envy her at all, her emotions, her friendships, the person she is striving to be all seem to be so problematic. I feel a great sense of relief at being able to say, "Well I've done what I've done with my life, I can't alter that, so I might as well get on and enjoy the rest."'

Many people have said that they can now see how their own bad judgment, lack of confidence, intransigence, fear, had a lot to do with the quality of their younger life. With maturity and self-knowledge they feel it may be possible to bring a different approach and new creativity to later life even though what they create then will never make up for misspent youth.

Jim, like many of the men who have spoken to me, went into a critical time in his forties because he felt he had failed to develop the creativity which was within him. He had worked, instead 'in the retail trade in different tedious jobs', he had children he hardly saw and felt his marriage was a trap. Once his children left home, his wife said she would go out to work and support him while he trained to be a furniture maker, giving him the chance to see if time ahead could be better than time past. 'It was wonderful,' he says. 'I loved the whole business of working with wood, I felt I had design ideas and I could make them work. I haven't done particularly well commercially but we manage, and I wake up feeling pleased to see the day, pleased with all the things which seemed to be a trap before.'

Judy, now in her forties, reflects on the first part of her life as a time which was in many ways difficult, painful and frustrating, but which has provided knowledge and experience she can now draw on. She explains: 'At a time when many others were knuckling down to careers, I was at least aware enough to know that I wasn't ready for the main work I had to do, and so I had jobs – all sorts – instead. Meanwhile I was insatiably curious, met lots of people, went to lots of places and was dogged by depression which I had to struggle to overcome time and again. At twenty-seven I met my husband and by thirty I had two children and a marriage that was failing. The breakdown of my marriage and of my health – I got tuberculosis – finally kick-started me and over the last years I have been moving out of that young, stuck state into a position where I feel more fluid and able to get down to work.

'Those transitional years have not been easy but at least there was movement and, I hope, growth. I've already experienced plenty of loss and I feel some of the mid-life grieving may have been done earlier, over what seemed for a long time a wasted youth. In fact I don't think that now. It's all been grist to the mill. In some ways I feel I have been privileged to have led this life. As I get older I can see the patterns created by the past and put them to use.

'I don't have the terror, professionally, of being superannuated as it seems so many people do. I haven't really started yet! I wonder if some of what people suffer isn't to do with having been around for a long time and being too familiar a figure to themselves. For me there's a great irony when people talk of being washed up at forty.'

In an overgrown Suffolk garden, swept by the East Anglian wind and visited occasionally by the resident Vietnamese pig, I talked with the writer Elspeth Barker, widow of poet George Barker. She was telling me of a life in which as a young, beautiful, innocent Canadian, swept off her feet by love, she was drawn into George Barker's complicated world which already included the writer Elizabeth Smart and her five children by him. Elliptically, she drew a picture of the years spent producing children and coming to grips with Barker's eccentric and unpredictable lifestyle. Fascinating and exhilarating years, but years in which she did not dare risk her own writing and putting her head above the parapet. But soon after he died she completed and published her first book, an exquisitely expressed and detailed novel *O Caledonia*. It promptly won a run of prizes. And there was Elspeth in her early fifties when we met, reflecting slightly wistfully on what had been, but also recognizing that at this time she was charting a path no less demanding than the one she had already trodden.

These thoughts she put to paper in an article for the *Observer*:

What the hell, Mehitabel? What of now? Now is as good and as ghastly as ever. I who have skulked on the peripheries and used most tricks to get out of the serious business of living. I am startled to find myself embarked on a strenuous new life with new sets of obligations ... I realize now that this is a fine time. I don't care about being young or old or whatever. I am past the anxieties of earlier days, no longer concerned about image or identity. At this interesting point in life, one may be whoever and whatever age one chooses ... One may also move very slowly round the garden in a shapeless coat, planting drifts of narcissus bulbs for later springs.

Those who can achieve this kind of rapprochement with themselves at mid-life are fortunate, but many of us still believe at some level that all the negative ideas we have imbibed about what it means to get older are the reality. We are not convinced by surveys and it is my belief that we must turn to the more personal affirmations which make real the notion of a fruitful later life. We may not buy the line of Robert Browning's Rabbi Ben Ezra who declared, 'The best is yet to be,' but we might be convinced by lesser but nevertheless optimistic suggestions.

In an extremely rare gesture of interest in what senior members of society have to say and get up to in their lives, the BBC produced their superb series 'The Nineties'. Here a group of spirited, mentally fine-tuned, adventurous and fascinating nonogenarians were given the opportunity to come across to the audience as real people – people who were old without being Golden Girls or the cast of 'One Foot in the Grave'. There was not a suggestion of patronage or caricaturing of the subjects. They were treated with a degree of seriousness that allowed us to take part in their lives, their passions and ideas and to have a real sense of lives worth living. There has also been a flurry of publishers bringing out books in Britain, the rest of Europe and America validating the ageing process – a response no doubt to the fact that the market for such books is growing as the bulge-and-boom generations begin to realize this is their concern. *I Don't Feel Old* and *Growing Old Disgracefully* are two invigorating and inspiring volumes of oral history which give fascinating insight into the worlds of their subjects, and they are a reminder of how important those who carry the history are as the last witnesses of their era in our so rapidly changing world. And we who have been such pioneers of change and who have been part of vastly shifting social mores, will have a fascinating oral history to pass down. Catherine Itzin and her co-writers of *I Don't Feel Old* saw themselves as playing their part in kicking against the stereotyping of older age, and in their introduction which is based on interviews with fifty-five men and women aged from sixty into their eighties, they explain their perspective: 'Contrary to the all too common belief that ageing is essentially an unavoidable process of retreat, of withdrawal into passivity and dependence, the truth is that for most men and women later life is a time of active challenge'.

The truth of those words are brought to life by 'Wayne Booth' who is in fact George M Pullman, Professor of English Emeritus at the University of Chicago. At the age of seventy-one he took on the subject of ageing in his book *The Art of*

Growing Older, a compilation of writings brought together with his own thoughts which shows the enormously varied ways in which people have tackled the business of ageing, some distinctly gloomy, while others are remarkably upbeat, although the over-riding message is of life-force, creativity, humour and grace. Booth sets out good reasons why we contemporary mid-lifers, slouching towards greater longevity than generations before us, should read it: 'Ageing in itself worries us moderns more than it worried our ancestors. They had other troubles to think about, especially the threat of early, painful, terrifying disease and death. They all had good reason to fear that they would die fairly soon. Why fear old age when early death was much more probable?'

As I made my way through his exploration of growing old, I became enchanted by this man, dazzled by the mind, the wit, the energy he exuded. And the fact that he is old enough to be my father (just) was manifestly a virtue. Like the nimblest of spinners he twirls together so many reflections, perceptions, curses and celebrations, on what his advancing years have meant that I found myself longing to sit down with him and hear his thoughts and hopefully believe that I too could experience the things which, he says, make older life a pleasure: 'Ripened friendship and deepening love, a laughter that depends on mature vision, a sense of freedom from the ills and limitations of youth, and a deepened capacity for religious contemplation and prayer ... NEW discoveries, not just compensations for what ageing inevitably subtracts.'

This picture of very old age being all about what the years have added is seen in the character of Pepe, who the author M. F. K. Fisher described in her book *Sister Age*, evoking such a feeling of beauty and vitality in his oldness. Written in the later years of her own life, she created some magical insights into ageing in this book. Of Pepe she wrote:

Every night he played bezique with his son, and at meals he pulled out my chair for me and served with ceremony and skill some special little dish he had bought on his long afternoon walk ... When meeting he bowed low over their [two young women's] hands and told them without a smile that he regretted having lost all but one tooth, because he liked to be 'well appointed' when he met charming ladies. Last time we saw him he was sitting on the stone wall of a bridge. He looked like Don Quixote, gaunt and old and still eager for new windmills to tilt at.

It is rare that old people are described with such delight and in a way that brings us, the outsider, to see dignity and something to be aspired to in the portrait. Rather we are dogged by the notion that each year we get older is about the lessening of what we are, that subtraction is precisely the sum of ageing. Seneca the Roman rhetorician might have been talking about the choice we face in how we will make the inevitable journey through mid-life: 'The fates lead him who will. He who won't they drag.' But if we need dragging it is perhaps because it is difficult to believe in serendipity when we think our journey is to join a group which has been effectively disenfranchised.

Much of the blame then lies with the vastly powerful image-making businesses designed to sell products which have pretty much ignored the elderly except when trying to sell pension schemes, laxatives and pipe tobacco, while the press has mostly dealt in tales of shock-horror treatment of our dear old folk, the horrors of granny dumping or the occasional sentimental tale of derring-do. No matter that older people watch at least as much television as younger people do, they are certainly not represented with the same diversity and interest value. Television has a limited repertoire of ideas on what ageing people are like and it is one of the things which has most raised the ire of my interviewees.

The approach is similar throughout Europe and America but it is only now that there are signs of change. It would be nice to believe these were a revolutionary recognition of the idea that older people may be as worthwhile as subjects for the public eye as their younger compatriots, but we should not delude ourselves. The reasons older people are beginning to creep into advertising, television programmes and films and to be included in surveys and reports of trends are simple. The first is that the image-making industries throughout the developed West are peopled with mid-lifers in positions of power. These are the talented, brash kids of the 1960s and 1970s who have grown up and one thing is sure – they are not going to acknowledge that they are getting too old to feature as part of the real world, part of the action and the script. So what better way to ensure that their stage in life comes to be seen as an attractive proposition than by having a few chic, eminently desirable middle-aged characters make their way into our daily visual fare?

It is par for the course in the view of Gary Thomas, a provincial journalist who recently turned fifty and whose wrinkled face and seriously grey hair bother him not a jot. He says: 'My generation and the one just behind have set the agenda throughout our lives. We are like the big gang on the street, leaders of the pack, and I am quite convinced it will go on happening. We'll be the generation to make old age the place to be, and we'll make sure we're noticed and respected for the knowledge and experience we have notched up. We're a bolshie lot and I don't see us quietly doffing our caps and saying, "Thanks for having me and now I'll settle into three or four decades of keeping out of everyone's way, tucked into my zimmer frame."'

The signs are certainly there that the bulge-and-boom generations will be targeted and made a good deal more visible than their predecessors have been. And if we accept that negative imagery is very effective in downgrading older age, then the encouraging flipside is that, if the imagery becomes positive, you never know, it just might make getting older look like the thing to do.

This is of course a mercenary trend, a direct bid for the so-called third-agers' disposable income, and going back to Neil Mackwood's *Sunday Times* article: 'On a purely demographic level, the Oldies have a significant advantage. There are 14 million people aged between fifty and seventy-four in Britain [this was in 1992]. They are the group with the highest disposable income ... making the baby-boomer generations of the 1940s and 1950s into the single most powerful demographic group.' And certainly if we are talking spending power, it is not surprising that the business world is schmoozing up to older generations. The figure for over-fifties in Britain alone, at the end of the 1980s, was put at £108 billion and was set to continue climbing. *Communique*, a publication for the European Year of Older People and Solidarity Between the Generations, talks of Britain's over-fifties as being the wealthiest in Europe and having the highest disposable income per capita. Michael Rybarski of the US based Age Wave which advises US industry on ageing, states that the over-fifties 'probably own about 80 per cent of all the wealth in the UK'.

A good chunk of this is tied up in property, but even so over-fifties are able to outspend younger consumers in many areas, so we are set to be a highly desirable section of society. There may be some amusement for us, in this scenario, as we watch to see how easily the admen and adwomen, who have honed their skills selling to the young and disdaining elders, get their approach right for those they so recently despised. It may not be so simple, opined Sue Pryke, writing in *Marketing Weekly*: 'Qualitative research into the over-fifties market reveals a huge discrepancy between marketers' views of older people and the self-image of many of the UK's healthier and wealthier recent retirers. For this is a new generation of "selfish oldies" discovering new freedoms, new priorities and above all the opportunity to behave badly.'

There is something instantly appealing about the idea that instead of being so boring we are ignored, we are instead getting the slightly racy tag of bad behaviour. What Pryke is saying here, is that they have an incautious, live-for-the-moment style. She notes that greys who have lived earlier years in a way they believed would win them respect and status in later life – abiding by a strong work ethic, showing loyalty to their firms and willingness to sacrifice personal pleasure and time in order to provide for the family – find this package undervalued by society. And, Pryke says, just as disaffected youth turns against the code of conduct assumed for it, so older people are being equally assertive. She explains: 'They are developing a mood of rebellion, usually on retirement, in which they can justify a spend-rather-than-save mentality, a shorter- rather than longer-term outlook, and a less conformist mentality. It is women who tend to have the most ambitious fantasies, breaking out from their mother and housewife role ... and the last thing this group see themselves as is old. If anything they feel younger than they have for years.'

If the industry has spotted more money available, they will certainly be looking for effective ways to persuade those who control the money to spend it. And you can be sure it means heavy seduction methods. Money talks in the consumer-led Western societies and throughout Europe and America, and the business world has begun to recognize that its own survival depends on finding some empathetic and enticing imagery and language for the nation's elders. Ben Evans, a planner with the advertising agency J. Walter Thompson, is well aware of the urgent need for a change. He shares the view that middle-aged people and elder people are stereotyped in adverts, often being made to appear older and more staid in body and attitude than they may be in reality. He says: 'Although life, attitudes and human behaviour has changed over recent years, images have not changed much in twenty years. But it is essential that we do better. The new greys are an extremely powerful and significant group and we haven't yet untangled who they are. So not only do we not understand the consumer, but we massively underestimate them. Advertising at present, for this group, is quite patronizing and narrow in its interpretation.'

But advertising is not the only industry which has turned its attention in a wholly new way towards a concern with the ageing population. An area which is growing constantly is anti-ageing science where boffins are conjuring extraordinary dreams of what may be possible, talking of the possibility of extending life by tens or even hundreds of years. Even without the race among scientists to create human life that will extend way beyond what nature ever intended, longevity has almost doubled in the past century, for those who have enjoyed a better standard of living, nutrition and health care and particularly in the years since the last war. And the number of people living to be one hundred in Britain rises steadily as we move towards the new millennium: in 1951 there were 300 people in Britain over the age of 100; by 1992 there were 6000 and in fifteen years' time it is calculated that more than 5 per cent of the population will be over eighty.

Amongst the best publicized ideas being explored are those of a leading physiologist at the University of Texas Health Science Center in San Antonio who believes that if dietary restriction, a method of increasing longevity which has been successfully tested on rodents, can have the same effect in humans, average life will be extended by some thirty years. In their laboratories Dr Michael Rose, at the University of California, and Dr Leon Luckinbill at Wayne State University in Detroit, have concentrated on looking at whether it may be possible to replicate what they are achieving with fruitflies. By selecting only the longest-living flies in a population then breeding them, then repeating this process over a six-year experimental period, life expectancy was upped by about one-third. The question is can this same approach be translated to the human species?

But the most pressing question at the core of the scientific work going on everywhere is why we age at all. If scientists can discover that, will they be able to prolong life indefinitely? American scientific journalists Ann Giudici Fettner and Pamela Weintraub have talked of ageing as 'the tragic side-effect of life'. They explain: 'The hormones released during puberty and as a result of stress slowly erode the body's organs. The food we eat and the air we breathe generate highly reactive free radicals, which make subtle but deadly changes in DNA. And environmental hazards from ordinary sunlight to industrial toxins, infiltrate the cells, helping to grind their engines to a halt. Some scientists have even found compelling evidence for an ageing clock in the brain. As that clock winds down, they say, it alters the levels of hormones and other biological substances, slowly lowering the effectiveness of the heart, lungs, immune system, and just about everything else that keeps the body healthy and strong.'

John Grimley Evans, Professor of Clinical Gerontology at Oxford University, talks of an interaction between genetic disposition and environment as the things which currently determine how long we live. He explains: 'You can't alter what is genetically determined without changing the genes, but how far you get towards your genetically determined maximum lifespan, and what disabilities you acquire along the way, can be controlled. As control of the environment has improved, so more people are living longer and I would put the maximum age at present at around 110 to 115 years' – others say 120 years is the maximum. Looking forward Professor Grimley Evans, a cautious prophet, believes that in, say, ten years, work on genes will make it possible to expand the maximum lifespan slighty.

Such caution is less apparent in American laboratories where molecular biologists are attempting to isolate the gene which leads to ageing and to explore how damage to the DNA may be prevented or reversed. Joan Smith-Sonneborn, Professor of Zoology and Physiology at the University of Wyoming, spoke to the American *OMNI* magazine about her work inducing damage in DNA cells with ultraviolet radiation, after which she photoreactivated them to help erase the damage. She discovered from this that the cells recovered and lived substantially longer than the never-damaged cells. There are enormous implications in this for human cells, she says, and talks of being close to a 'major breakthrough'.

We can be forgiven, as we contemplate a normal lifespan

which we might expect to be stretched by five or ten years beyond what our forebears had, for feeling unnerved at the sci-fi talk of the anti-ageing competitors who, a bit like Las Vegas gamblers, conjecture who will be able to add on the largest number of years – some talk of 100 or even 200 extra years being added on to life. The quest for limitless longevity fuels the dreams of people like David Brown, an original member of the Alliance for Ageing and the founder of the Foundation for the Enhancement and Extension of Life (FEEL) in America who is quoted as saying: 'A thousand years sounds good to me.'

The first reaction is to laugh, but if we consider that scientists may well come to a way of achieving some kind of greatly extended longevity in time, it is vital that we stop to consider whether this is really desirable. Imagine if we were to live just fifty or a hundred extra years, what problems it would pose for other generations, for governments attempting to finance society's needs. It is an idea which raises enormous questions of ethics and we, as the potential subjects of all this, should be addressing them. We need to ask whether we consider it morally acceptable to become latter-day Methuselahs, to choose to have life extended in an already over-crowded world where projections for the population explosion into the next century are dire. What would it mean in a world where resources are already being used up far too rapidly, if those of us who could afford to – and the likelihood is that longevity *would* become just another commodity to be bought unless it could in some way be pre-programmed for everyone – decided we wanted to double or triple our lifespan? It is not difficult to imagine how it would upset an already very fragile ecological balance and endanger our children's generation.

It all brings to mind people wishing to be frozen so that they may come back to life at some future time, or the American organization The Immortalists where members sincerely believe that, through mind over matter, they can keep themselves alive indefinitely. There is something terrifying in this desire for omnipotence, the belief that we have the right to never-ending tenure in this life. Far better, in my view, is to endeavour to find a way to live our lives which are, anyway, naturally extended further than ever before, in the best and most fulfilling way possible.

Finding the best way to live our lives and then to prepare for our death is the aim of the Omega Institute, a recently set up think-tank with a New Age approach which, based in America, aims to look at constructive ways of ageing. It has drawn together gerontologists, physicians, psychologists, sociologists, anthropologists, philosophers, ethicists, cultural observers and spiritual leaders. Dr Stephen Rechtshaffen, director of the Institute, is one of the large team who believe we are moving towards defining ageing in a different way. He talks of 'Conscious Ageing' as the way the new cultural elite is presenting it and explains: 'This is a new way of looking at and experiencing ageing that moves beyond our cultural obsession with youth toward a respect and need for the wisdom of age.' In other words it is a group of people who have come to see what has been lost in cultures where youth has been the gold standard and where we have lost sight of the hierarchy of status and value which people have in many parts of Asia and Africa as they age. A hierarchy through which the knowledge and wisdom acquired through grappling with the complex practical, emotional and psychological tasks of life, is passed down as valuable learning. I have seen this at work in African rural communities where the elders who have spent years growing their food can teach their juniors, just as in Sri Lanka I saw the fishermen, grave old men who had spent many years fishing the waters, showing young men where to go, how best to tempt the fish. In return, and quite naturally, youngers respect them for their knowledge, just as older women in many developing countries are seen to have spiritual wisdom and they are seen as able to help younger people with their problems.

But how many of us in the West have turned, in our

growing years, to elders to learn something, to try to understand our troubled inner worlds? Very few I suspect. The hallmark of the post-war years is that we have handed over all these tasks to experts. Teachers drum knowledge into us, instructors impart skills, psychologists, counsellors and therapists are there to help us grapple with our inner confusions. Where in the midst of all this is there a place for the older person's knowledge and wisdom to be passed down? How often do youngsters think for an instance that their grandparents might be the people who could be of value?

Not often, although when it happens it can be an enriching experience. Irene Oliver, who is in her seventies, and grandmother to Joe describes how, when Joe was studying for an exam in modern history, she was able to help: 'I trawled up all my memories and just talked with Joe about how the war years had been, what we had done, how we felt, the broadcasts we remembered . . . He told me how it had brought everything to life for him and made it far easier to visualize and remember than if he'd just had books to read.'

Anne Eade who shares the house with her daughter and son-in-law, and is visited daily by her granddaughter Daisy, is forever discussing her way of doing things and the past with Daisy, comparing it with what happens these days. She says: 'Daisy takes a lot of interest in what I say and in a way we have an exchange. I love hearing about her life and she seems to like hearing about mine. I would say we respect each other because we can see what each other has to offer, and that's the way I think it should be.'

Can an organization like the Omega Institute reinstate respect and affection for age at a time when generations seem to be ever more distant from each other, where hostilities and alienation are a constant topic of conversation? There is a will for it to happen but has the divide between generations become so entrenched that, unless we consider how it could be otherwise, and actively look for ways to re-create some of the interaction between generations which existed in earlier times,

it is unlikely to happen? Answering questions for the Eurobarometer survey the vast majority of people throughout the
European member states said they would like to see more links
between the older and younger generations. But Hannah Eadie,
now in her seventies, founder of the Positive Ageing Project
has found, she says, 'a lot of older people so down on the
young . . . terribly intolerant', and she sees it as a loss for
everyone. This is something we should listen to for we, at mid-
life are in a position to alter a pattern of living and communicating that has separated older and younger generations in such a
way that communication, let alone respect is often gone
altogether.

Tackling this damaging and saddening schism is the aim of
various organizations which have set up cross-generational
schemes, and which draw inspiration from the kind of societies
discussed where skills are passed down. The Dark Horse
Venture, a wonderfully imaginative, broad-based project which
aims to stimulate over-fifty-fives to develop interests, and
involve themselves in a huge range of activities, including
volunteer work, has a generations-working-together scheme.
The idea here, explains founder Mary Thomas, is to find ways
in which a person with a lifetime of skills and experience can
offer some of this to younger people in a school, planning
activities with a group of younger people, helping them with
homework or in making a model for example. 'The aim is to
develop a relationship as well as to share skills,' she explains.
Creating relationships is at the heart of Age Concern's new
Trans Age initiative, based on the United States' successful
Foster Grandparent Programme. Here older volunteers are
recruited from every class and ethnic background, to work
with young children with critical needs at family centres,
hospitals and crèches. 'Magic Me', the scheme in the inner-city
borough of Tower Hamlets in London inspired by the pioneer-
ing work done in Baltimore, gives older people a role as
mentors with children. Taking part in programmes of shared
creative activities such as photography, music-making, dancing

and story-telling, school children and older people living in residential homes, hospitals and shared housing schemes get to know each other well.

But there is an irony not to be missed in this quest of ours for respect and reverence when it was we who most effectively denied the validity of age for our own parent generation. It is a situation on which Janet Daley, columnist for *The Times*, has remarked: 'In my parents' generation, there was some authority and veneration attached to ageing. To be young still meant being callow, untried and unwise. When John Major and I (and Neil Kinnock and Norman Lamont and Howard Brenton and Baroness Blackstone and Paul McCartney and all those who are now around fifty) were striplings in the 1960s, the young had usurped moral authority from their elders. Even the political leaders of the day – John Kennedy in the United States and Harold Wilson in Britain – were uncommonly youthful and both had taken over from exceptionally fusty predecessors. Not to be young then meant being a know-nothing.'

Then the irony on top of this original irony is that, at mid-life, like at no other time, we need our elders to look to. We are suddenly like kids who have been allowed all the permissiveness in the world to run wild, but now we have reached the point where being allowed to make the rules doesn't look such fun any more. The future is a *tabula rasa* and what we need is to see, hear and know inspiring role models. We need to be able to turn as Susan does to Lois, who is thirty years her senior, and see 'a person who I admire so much because she seems to understand so much that I don't, so when I am making a decision I visit and discuss it, when I am down I turn to her because she seems to have a wonderfully seasoned perspective, when I am happy she celebrates with me in the most generous way'. It brings us back to the importance of shifting our own values and prejudices in order to see the many and varied elders who can offer inspiration.

Simone de Beauvoir, who loathed the idea of ageing as

much as anyone, and had no wish to acknowledge that it would be her fate, nevertheless saw clearly the importance of finding role models: 'We must stop cheating: the whole meaning of our life is in question in the future that is waiting for us. If we don't know what we are going to be, we cannot know what we are: let us recognize ourselves in this old man or in that old woman. It must be done if we are to take upon ourselves the entirety of our human state.'

And what of friendship at mid-life? It is a time when many of us see friends as becoming increasingly important, the bonus in having more freedom as children go and perhaps work diminishes. In the young adult years, all too often friends with whom we have been very close while growing up, become sidelined as we settle with partners, have families, become absorbed in work and perhaps a social life connected with it, and here we are at a time when the possibilities for the friendships to be nurtured, to grow and be a place we support each other in the next part of our journey, are exciting.

A couple of years ago I took a two-week trip to America, with a woman friend I have known for more than twenty years. Through the years we have seen each other spasmodically, spoken on the phone a certain amount, but there was always the sense that things must be curtailed, there was no time to meet or even chat as fully as we would have liked. Quite gradually as my children became more absorbed in their lives, less eager to fill mine, I began to see this friend – and others – for weekend walks, for an evening out and our telephone conversations became more frequent and longer. It was as though a space was opening out for this friendship so that there was a place where we could discuss what was happening in our lives, we could share how it felt to be growing older, the problems for her of having an ageing mother. There was time for the intimacy which had always been there, but at a low level, to spread and strengthen. When we decided we would like to make the trip together we found the time. Her children had left home, mine were pretty independent; my partner accepted that I wanted to spend some time with a friend, that although I value my relationship with him, my friendships too are important in a different way. I find that as I age I become clearer about not having to tailor down these important friendships because I live with a partner, because it is social convention that one does not go on holidays without one's partner.

We had a glorious time, talking in the close, life-exploring way women do. We drew on our history, giggled a great deal, played counsellor to each other when, suddenly, some buried pain or problem surfaced. In this time our friendship moved beyond what it had been when we were younger women. It became a new, deeper friendship, a product of our maturity.

The value of friendship as we age is that, at a time when life may appear to be shrinking, it extends it and feeds it and it is the sense of being bound up with others who matter to you and to whom you matter.

Friendships may revolve around domestic matters, bringing up children, our relationships with partners, whereas as we move into the new life-stage in which we may no longer be so absorbed in these matters, the quality of friendships can alter. They may grow and embrace more philosophical and intellectual concerns. This is how it has been for Julia: 'Nothing has been planned differently, my close friends are the people I have met around the children, mostly, but I find now that when they come to have coffee, or we go out for a meal, we are much more likely to discuss our views on life, on politics, on things we are reading. It is as though we are growing up together, recognizing that there is a new time in which we can share these wonderful stimulating things, a time in which we can reach further out into the world and share what we find. It's quite thrilling and unexpected.'

For Bob it is happening around his hobby, motorbiking. The years until now – he is in his mid-fifties – have been spent working hard at his factory job, being at home with his wife and daughters and seeing 'mates at the pub' but that, he says firmly, was not about 'real friendship'. With the motorbike club which he attends most weekends, now his children have left home, he finds a camaraderie with fellow bikers and out of that has grown a closeness and companionship he values. He says: 'I find if something is bugging me, if I'm worried, if I'm upset one of the men – there are only four of us – will spot it and somehow he gets me talking and that always makes me feel better. I do it for them as well and I feel that we really know each other quite well and I value the time with them. I see it as an important part of my life.'

To Ethel friends are the fabric of a day-to-day existence in the small town where she lives: 'Molly's a great friend. She rings me up and says come and have a drink and we have one together and a chat, then next time it's my turn. Then there's another Molly who's a painter and we talk about that. Nancy is one of my oldest friends and we have a lot of fun. My friends are all different but it is knowing they are all there, as part of my life, that they are my world, that matters.' June Barraclough, now half-way through her mid-life years, feels similarly: 'Friends of one's own generation are invaluable as one grows older, their price above rubies.'

The importance of people who are close, who understand us, care for us and who in return can accept our caring for them was what Simone de Beauvoir, who invested much in friendship, put in a way worth hearing: 'One's life has value so long as one attributes value to the life of others, by means of friendship.' In a more prosaic way the value of a nurturing reciprocity is shown in research where the writers talked of how mortality as well as morbidity is reduced in ageing people through 'expressive and caring' relationships including friendship.

In hearing what older people have to say, those of us who have not thought about friends as of particular importance in later life, may see what it can mean. Winston, in his seventies, who came to Britain from the Caribbean as a young man, talks of 'the importance of perhaps ten close peers who have been with me through the painful times, as when my wife died, who know me well enough that I can be quite relaxed with them. I can laugh when I want and cry when I want.'

Mary Gwinnell says: 'Friends are central to my life. I have one friend from infant school days and I write to her once or twice every week. I visit her for three days or so two or three times a year. When I moved to my present home I made a determined effort to find friends, even hobbling out the gate and accosting a likely-looking woman walking a dog – she turned out to be the daughter of an earl. We became friends and have remained close. Making friends in later life is no different from those made earlier on and I have a friend twenty years older than I am and friends among my mature students – last year four of them took to coming to dinner and spending the evening watching my videos of operas.'

Women traditionally have shared intimacy, have talked about feelings, and so have tended to maintain the important friendships made during life's different stages. Feminism has drawn many of us together over the past three decades, linking us through politics and passion, but also through sharing problems and pains. Women who have been abused, who have felt themselves hopeless and helpless in their relationships or jobs, have formed friendships which, once the crisis has passed, often flower into entertaining, life-enhancing bonds. Women's shared experiences have led us to see how valuable we are to each other. Mary Dubuffet, an activist in the early years of the women's movement, speaks for many women when she describes the changes she feels feminism has made to women's lives, in bringing them close to each other and building a valued trust and intimacy. She recalls a home life in which women friends played no part: 'My mother despised women and still does and although this was not how all women felt about others, I think, before feminism, there was a lot of ambivalence – women were nice as mates but they were also competition. Then there was the attitude I had when much younger, that most women were airheads.

'It is terrible to admit now, but I was very bright and very successful academically and in truth I had a low view of most women who seemed to me not to be matching men in the world. I then became involved with feminism because the politics so clearly made sense to me and it was through this that I was able to see women for the first time in all their three-dimensional-ness and to make wonderful, enduring friendships. My husband could not understand it when I told him that the feelings I would have if one of my closest friends died, would not be different from him dying. Yet when she did die recently it was just that kind of loss, and I feel it now as something which will be missing in my life ahead. But in the same way the friends who are around are precious to me and I know that they will be, if anything, more so in years ahead, and so I give them time and energy.

'Women are the people in whose hands I have placed my emotional safety and care. I am single now and I feel if I have a nervous breakdown, as nearly happened recently when a number of shocking and painful things happened in quick succession, if I am ill, if in some way I cannot cope, there are women who understand and can support and help me as I would them. Yet we live in a society which doesn't really encourage us to understand that friends are as vital as anyone or anything else in our lifetime.'

American film director Linda Yellon recognizes that she has made a painful choice in dedicating her time and energy so thoroughly to film-making, that she has reached her forties without a partnership or, more significantly, children. She sat on a bar stool in the LA café where we met, an attractive, spirited woman, talking frankly and intimately. With what seemed admirable integrity she acknowledged that her life is so bound up with work it would be difficult for her to make enough space for children, that she might well not have juggled career and family successfully.

Instead she has developed deep and important friendships, some with men but most significantly with women and it was this that she celebrated at the age of forty by making *Chantilly Lace*, a film 'about a woman turning forty as I was, and who wanted to share it with her circle of friends away at a house in the country for a weekend. I wanted the film to be about truth, about how women relate because that is, to me, one of the most important things we have in life.'

She explains how it evolved: 'I had a script of what, broadly, should happen but the dialogue was created organically, by the actresses, as they played out the story and felt how they would behave. It was an extraordinary experience because I really felt it showed the relationship that women can have with each other, and it opened up feelings of the woman getting older in a society where that is so hard.

'Because it was my own story too I was very involved and the thing that came out most powerfully was how for women friendship is the most enduring aspect of their lives. They would go through relationships with parents, relationships with lovers, and in the centre of all that friendship was the grounding area, the place of solace and secure love when they needed that.'

It is here that women seem so much luckier than men. Men do have close friendships but they tend to be more constrained, more guarded, often more competitive than women's close friendships. Their culture has not made it easy or seemingly normal to develop friendships as intimate, openly loving and supportive as women's. They may indeed be close, but rather as tortoises might be close, with an impenetrable shell protecting the soft part. This kind of friendship is exemplified in Anita Brookner's *A Private View*, a tale of George and Michael who were devoted friends but allowing devotion to be as nurturing or protective as it could have been, was beyond the rules of male friendship. John Bayley summed it up in his review (*Spectator* 18 June 1994): 'They worked for the same firm; they had retired more or less together; and they had planned together to take a long leisurely trip to the Far East. Further than that their togetherness does not go and had never been.'

This level of deep companionship is certainly of great value to men when they find time, conviction and courage to foster it. Anthony Trollope expresses as well as anyone what this means to men in his novel *The Warden*. With wonderful understatement he writes: 'The Bishop and Mr Harding loved each other warmly – they had grown old together – they were all in all to each other.'

At least in the war days men grew up in circumstances where, however tightly the upper lip might have been held, there were times when it wobbled and collapsed so that feelings, fears and problems were shared. But the post-war days have done much to destroy opportunities for male friendship. The all-boys public school system which has boomed during these years, may thrust the chaps together but all too often it also teaches them very thoroughly that male friendships should be of the locker-room variety, all tough talk and plenty of machismo, and that tears and softness are not the stuff of manhood. The world of work has become increasingly pressurized and for the majority of men the pressures to make their mark, progress up the ladder, bring home the bacon, have been sufficiently great to allow little time for the kind of friendship which needs space and relaxedness to develop.

It is something Vic Seidler, author of *Men, Sex and Relationships* has felt to be a dreadful deprivation in men's lives. He has, in middle life, involved himself in setting up men's groups to explore the emotional issues in their lives which so often are a taboo subject.

Camaraderie at work, playing sports together, going out for a drink and a chat, are all thoroughly acceptable, but Vic says: 'If men touch on anything that really matters to them inside, they are likely to be regarded as weird, weak and not masculine. If they talk emotionally to another man they are likely to be branded as gay and backed away from. The prohibition on men's emotions, from such a very young age, does not make it easy for them to open up to each other, to form the kind of nurturing relationships women have. I have been very envious of women, watching what feminism has given them, and out of that grew my determination to work in a similar way with men. It has certainly been worth it, I do have male friends with whom I can share the deepest feelings and vice versa and that has added something very important to my life.'

We need to encourage men, as they need to encourage themselves, to look at how in mid-life they might start building friendships, forming bonds and links which could do a great deal to lessen the horror of retirement. Perhaps as this happens earlier for many and as the activeness and confidence of the middle-years are extended into the seventies, as is now pro-jected, men will find the time to create, build and nurture friendships. Perhaps the example of feminism, and of what Bob describes as 'the enviable closeness I see in women and its absence in my own life', will set men on course to take the risk of intimacy among themselves. It is what Bob has in mind when he says: 'I think I haven't valued friendship enough with men or with women, and it is something I am trying now to change.'

Perhaps if this kind of shift takes place, men will be able to love and mourn their friends openly, rather than resorting to the droll understatement to disguise their pain as Logan Pears-all Smith does: 'I cannot forgive my friends for dying: I do not find these vanishing acts of theirs at all amusing.'

The friendships we have with our own gender are not, of course, the only kind we may have made through the years, and plenty of us find something particular and valuable in being able to understand through a friend of the opposite sex how their gender works in the world at large. Or the friendship may be very similar to those we have with women. Certainly this is how it is for Martin Bevan, now reaching fifty, who met the woman he regards as 'a friend I cherish' ten years ago. He is with a partner, she is married, but they have doggedly insisted on maintaining the friendship even when that has been problematic with their partners. Martin explains: 'Marianne, who is slightly older than I am, understands emotions and the games adults play with each other far better than any man I have met and I enjoy her company because it is feminine. We have never been sexually attracted but I would thoroughly enjoy spending more time with her, perhaps even sharing a house if we were both on our own.'

Maritza Jones is fifty-nine, a single parent, and since her children left home she 'nose-dived' at the awful feeling of being abandoned, 'the person left alone in an empty space while my kids went on to get completely involved in their lives'. She says: 'It was just chance that Peter, somebody I have known through work for years, came to the town where I was living the weekend I felt particularly bleak. I just poured everything out and he was extraordinarily understanding and said many useful things. I suppose that created a new intimacy between us because he then told me about his life and by the time he left that weekend our friendship had become something much more than it had been. The important thing was not to let it fade down again, and we both made the effort to phone regularly, write letters and we see each other quite regularly. Peter is important to me in the way women friends are.'

If there is a single issue on which most of us agree, it is that the state of our health is all-important to the quality of later life. The fear of being ill or finding our bodies fading down into painful inactivity is expressed time and again and I cannot count how often people have said they would not want greater longevity if they were not fit. Yet it is remarkable how many of us turn our eyes from the vast amounts of literature which spell out how we can lose weight, maintain a weight that is good for us, avoid cluttering up our hearts with cholesterol, damaging heart, lungs and just about everything else with cigarettes and stressing out our livers with alcohol, rather than acknowledge that there are ways we may take control of our health. Instead we all too often cling to the myths which tell us that bodies become weightier with each decade that we age and this is inevitable, that we mustn't over-exert ourselves as we get older, that doing what comes naturally, even if that means eating three immensely rich meals a day and then taking a bus to the cinema, is the right way to go.

One of the things doctors stress is that fifty is an important time for our health. We may feel older than we wish to be, but we are still young enough to choose how fit our bodies will be in later life. Professor Grimley Evans, whose lean, supple physique tells more clearly than any words what the late fifties can look like, takes a firm line on the need to take responsibility for our health telling us: 'Middle age is a good time for people to make a formal appraisal of their lifestyle and face the future with confidence and determination rather than the sense of despair that afflicts some of us. I think every year or so one should reappraise one's dietary habits, alcohol intake, smoking, exercise and so on . . .' He is in good company, for there is increasing evidence that those of us who are overweight, out of condition and beginning to feel less well than in earlier years can reverse this situation by learning that we need less food, because our metabolism slows as we age. But we must eat the right kind of food. Doctor Richard Hochschild at the Hoch Company in California has looked into the things that affect whether our chronological age is higher or lower than what is described as our 'body age' – that is determined to some extent, at least, by how we look after ourselves. He spelled out, in an article in the *Daily Mail*, just how thoroughly what we eat makes its mark, explaining that ten servings of high-fat food a day will age an average forty-five-year-old man by six years; a woman who eats fish and chicken rather than red meat is likely to be four biological years younger than her red-meat-eating counterpart. And those are some of many examples. Researchers at Bart's Hospital have found that reducing the amount of fat in the average British diet by one-sixth can cut blood cholesterol by 16 per cent which would prevent half of all heart attacks among men and women aged forty and one-fifth among those aged seventy. Over 100 studies have found that the amount of fruit and vegetables we eat has an impact on protecting against cancer.

Exercise can do as much as diet to reverse the trouble we may be storing up in our overweight, understretched bodies and the difference between the ever-growing number of middle-aged people who attend gyms, run the marathon, swim many lengths a day and play demanding sports and not only look wonderful but talk with delight about how fit they feel, and those who cannot or will not do much more than walk the dog around the block, is very visible. But much more significantly they may be buying their own longevity. There are experts in the field of ageing who believe regular, demanding exercise can offset heart disease; one piece of research suggested that regular aerobic exercise can take as much as ten years off the ageing of the heart. Studies in the USA and Sweden show that by taking only a gentle exercise programme, people of seventy, eighty and even ninety were able to increase their muscle bulk and strength by up to 100 per cent.

It may not be that easy taking our bodies in hand at mid-life – certainly Bill Cosby, who surveyed his body with horror as he reached fifty, did not think so: 'All the assorted parts of me used to be flat and hard; but in these twenty years of going downhill, I have seen the growth of a gut, the thickening of thighs, the emergence of flab.' But he started watching what he ate, developed a mean game of tennis and found his body leaner, his fitness level magically improved. But taking control of our bodies is not just about aesthetics; it is, in the view of Professor Grimley Evans and many, many others, about taking control of life itself. He is convinced that disability and disease are not inevitable consequences of ageing, but often the consequences of turning away from learning important mid-life lessons.

It is a lesson we are beginning to learn and take to heart. The voices of men and women who have come to what they describe as the moment of reckoning at mid-life, tell time and again of the curious pleasure they have found when they have taken themselves in hand. Women, particularly, tend to recognize as the last child leaves home, or they go out to work and a new routine is imposed on life, that they have slipped into bad and slothful habits and have not had the motivation to do anything about it.

Sally is one of these: 'I was on my own with my three kids and, even when they got into their teens, I would eat the same food as them – lots of stodge very often – and too much of it. I convinced myself I was getting lots of exercise Hoovering the stairs and putting washing into the machine. Then when the kids all went off to college I took a cool look at my health: I was a stone and a half overweight, I couldn't run for three minutes without thinking I'd die, and I seemed to have unaccountable aches and pains. My doctor was very clear about it: she told me I had the choice between ageing rather rapidly from now on, and finding myself at sixty able to do very little, or I could lose weight, start exercising and probably be a vigorous seventy-year-old. In other words there was nothing wrong with me that was beyond my control.' She took control, lost weight and, more importantly she feels, learned how to make bargains with herself so that she could over-eat on special occasions, binge once in a while, then 'sort it out' on another day.

Faced with a midriff which seemed, like Topsy, to grow and grow and more fatigue than seemed reasonable for his age, George Ball, a fifty-five-year-old social worker, cut down on alcohol, stopped eating puddings ('an awful sacrifice') and became a diet-book junkie: 'When I got bored with the approach in one I would keep myself on course by switching to a different "amazing diet method" – they all seemed to add up to much the same – and that way I knocked my midriff back and also managed to find a way of eating that keeps me full and doesn't fatten me.' He has taken up squash and yoga and has a protective attitude to his body now: 'I'm damned if I'm going to have a miserable old age because my body's been badly serviced. I wouldn't do that to my car, and – not before time – I've come to see that my body is rather more valuable.'

Getting to grips with physical health is relatively uncomplicated, even if it takes a profound effort of will, but there seems
no such way of protecting ourselves against what many of us
feel is the inevitability of losing mental and creative faculties.

We only need to look at the number of famous intellectuals,
artists of all kinds, professionals, entrepreneurs, craftspeople
and conversationalists who have carried on at full mental pitch
into their eighties and nineties to see that it is certainly not
inevitable. And there is work done by Wayne Dennis, Professor
of Psychology at Brooklyn College in America, into creative
productivity, which underscores the anecdotal belief that age
does not necessarily mean we cease to be able to use our
intellect as we did when younger. Indeed this research showed
that a higher percentage of the work done by historians,
philosophers and scholars was produced between sixty and
seventy than between twenty and thirty, while the productivity
of scientists kept a pretty straight level through the early to
middle years, declining a very small amount towards the
seventies. Ken Dychtwald in his setting-an-agenda-for-ageing
book, *Agewave* sums up research and says: 'Of the 30 million
Americans over the age of sixty-five, only 10 per cent show
any significant loss of memory and fewer than half of those
show any serious mental impairment.' Something similar was
found in a study published in 1995 by Harvard University
psychologist, Douglas Powell, author of *Profiles of Cognitive
Ageing* where tests were carried out on 1583 people aged from
twenty-five to ninety-two. More than 25 per cent of subjects in
their eighties performed as well as younger people and some
outstripped all age groups in such subjects as reading, compre-
hension and mathematics. Nearly one-third of people, he also
found, retain lucidity in their later years.

Although how far we disintegrate mentally is not entirely in
our hands, work from the University of California found that
lifelong mental activity can partially halt the process of deterioration of the brain. The belief is, explained psychologist Arthur
Shimamura, that, as with muscles in the body, the brain needs

exercise. Certainly it appears that older people who keep their minds occupied, stimulated, vigorous, do not appear to deteriorate as quickly as those who assume they can no longer learn or remember well.

Dr Joan Gomez tells us:

Since the mid-1980s research has provided clear evidence that age alone does not cause mental decay. Unless you allow dry rot to set in you can go on mastering new concepts well into your mid-eighties – avoiding rot to the brain involves exactly the same concerns with diet, cutting out damaging substances and taking exercise which brings oxygen to the brain, as caring for the body does. It also means providing the mind with stimulus, new challenges and a reason to, metaphorically speaking, keep its muscle tone intact.

This may cheer those of us who share the feeling of writer Claude Hartz that we have so much still to do and will happily exercise brain as well as body if we can help ourselves by doing so. He says: 'I feel I have only just learned, in my fifties, to write as I want so I'd like to live long enough to do all the things I have in mind. But that is the point: my mind must be up to it or there's no point at all and I'm careful about keeping my body fit as the engine which makes my mind work.'

And Mary Gwinnell, nearing her mid-seventies, is a very good example of the possibility Dr Gomez suggests. She made up for having left school at sixteen by deciding at the age of fifty, having reared four children, to get the education she missed earlier. She won a mature state scholarship and became an undergraduate at University College after which she was invited to do research which led to a Ph.D. She then took a teaching job in a girls' grammar school and has worked since, teaching and giving private tuition.

She reflects: 'I think I have fulfilled my potential intellectually and lived life the way I wanted. It is always a shock when I look in the mirror because I am unavoidably old, and I want to shout I am young, vital, growing intellectually and spiritually because that is how I feel, and I believe old people can remain interesting by going on growing; never losing a sense of wonder; being capable of being profoundly moved.'

Could anyone doubt that the mental faculties of Sir Geoffrey Jellicoe are not equal to those of men a quarter his age? Rather they seem to have matured and improved with experience. He has seen his landscape architecture practice grow bigger and more demanding than ever in the years between eighty and ninety-four and in 1994 was busy working on the massive Atlanta Historical Gardens in Georgia project. His legs are frail now and he stays indoors most of the time, but his mind works with as much agility as ever. Indeed his later years have seen a flowering of his creativity – he spoke of taking up drawing again (having dropped it at a younger age) when he was eighty and his pictures have since been exhibited at the Royal Academy.

We see far more clearly than our parent generation had the chance to do, battered as so many were by wars and hardship, lives preoccupied with finding a way of survival, what a spiritual support, a reinforcement of identity, a private strength, using our creativity can be. We hear this in the voice of poet and writer Adrienne Rich at the age of sixty-five saying that her creative energy shows no sign of waning: 'We get so much better as we get older'.

It was a quest to develop a creativity which had been suggested in earlier years but never given scope, which took Clarissa Beothy to art school in her early fifties. She is a Hungarian refugee, who came to Britain in her forties and she met a man with whom she has since lived. But with no personal outlet, she felt herself 'shrinking away' as she got older and she talked of how she often feared the emptiness of the future. In her early fifties she 'took a wild shot' and applied to the art college in Cornwall where she lives, to do a degree course. She had painted a small amount in the past but had no confidence in her abilities.

She recalls: 'When the letter came accepting me I was amazed, so thrilled, I went around for three days with nothing but a big smile. Then there was the reality of being in a class with much younger people, having to find a way to communicate with them which took time. But when it happened wonderful friendships were formed; the younger people seemed to see that, through the life I had lived, I had something valuable that they could learn from, and I learnt about how to be youthful again, in a way which hadn't been part of my life for a time.

'Physically it was tough because I didn't have the stamina they had to stand for hours at an easel, to work with clay and all the other physical work. It was hard, there were times when I wondered if I could keep up, but it was exciting . . . so exciting to be learning and developing.'

She went on to win an educational scholarship to go to Eastern Europe and to make a film about how the collapse of Communism was affecting artists. She says simply: 'My life has been transformed by all this. I have a heart to my existence, a form of expression which I want to go on using. My mid-life has certainly been a turning point, I see only that things will be better than in the past.'

The belief that having a sense of purpose is vital if we are to feel positive about ageing comes through loud and clear in the voices of mid-lifers. Alice Bryan began studying psychoanalysis at fifty and plans to train in Zurich; Robert Bryan quit his job as an engineer and got a job working at a scuba diving club, where he has been able to put to use a lifelong hobby; Susan Strachan, in mid-life, began training as a herbalist and went on to work with patients over fifty-five with chronic illness; Linda left a nursing job after the years spent bringing up a son to begin training as a counsellor; while David Lyons has cut back the time spent working to make time for regular writing, since the course he attended.

Education is something many older people talk of as the thing which banished loneliness and a sense of futility and the University of the Third Age, which has been set up across Europe since it was started in the UK by Peter Laslett, has offered learning, friendship and a sense of purpose to people who felt there was nowhere they would fit in to study. Others take degrees wherever possible with determination to take a path they have chosen.

Marie, an actress who ended her marriage when the children left home, is taking a degree in Third World studies and intends to work in the field in Africa. Will, a jewellery salesman, used his savings to study to become a probation officer in his mid-forties and is inclined to proselytize because he is so pleased by the decision. Others study simply because they want to acquire more knowledge. The level of zest and enthusiasm these people display in having a sense of purpose and being active is conspicuous, echoing the sentiments of Sir John Harvey-Jones who, at seventy, said: 'The day you stop flapping your wings is the day you fall off your perch.'

The prospect of ageing is more daunting for those whose own parents have become ill, have died too young or in a state of suffering, or as Jim describes of his parents: 'They seemed to settle into feeling cheated by life, being bitter and determined not to get anything out of life.' But far more frequent are the stories of inspirational parents whose zest for life and clear enjoyment of it are models for their own future. Cec Darker sums it up well, describing her own mother, now eighty: 'I have only just been able to keep pace with her as she strides across the hills. Put it this way, when I was doing twenty-five thousand things she seemed to be doing twenty-six thousand. I recently travelled with her to China after my father died and she was so full of interest in everything, so spirited and unfailingly courteous that absolutely everyone on the trip talked about how wonderful she was.'

The first half of life may embody some of the most dynamic and challenging events and opportunities, the significant tasks of adulthood. But an immensely rewarding counter-balance to that, as we see time and again in writings and poetry, and as has been expressed over and over to me, is enjoying the things to be done in life but also finding a tranquillity, a sense of internal peace, an acceptance of oneself. Anne Morrow Lindbergh, in her exquisite soliloquy on mid-life ('Gift From the Sea') written during days spent alone at a house near the sea, expresses the recognition of what was needed and her determination to reach it: 'I want to be at peace with myself. I want a singleness of eye, a purity of intention, a central core to my life . . . an inner harmony . . . which can be translated into outward harmony. This is an end towards which we could strive – to be the still axis within the revolving wheel of relationships, obligations and activities.'

Early in the 1990s *Time* magazine referred to us, the current generation of mid-lifers, as the Command Generation. Bernice Neugarten at Chicago University took this article as a starting point for questioning her mid-life research subjects to see if they did indeed feel in command. Her findings showed, she says, a new level of composure and competence in generations which have cut their teeth as pioneers. But although being pioneer mid-life generations has, quite clearly, many virtues, that doesn't mean we should minimize the very real challenge we face in making our way onwards from the middle years. Looked at positively, it is a wonderful opportunity to do and experience much that would be impossible in the shorter span generations before have had. But it is also daunting and the best way, I believe, to face the future with confidence and optimism, is to look forward at the best of what there is in later life.

Two very different anecdotes which seem to me to show how varied our roles and satisfactions may be, appeal to me particularly. Tassaduq Ahmed reflects on seventy-one years, during which he was involved in a youth movement 'against colonial domination' in East Pakistan and, since coming to Britain, he has worked with and for Bengali people in the East End of London where he lives, telling with pride that he is now chair of the Spitalfields Small Business Association. Like many older people I have spoken with, Tassaduq has no wish to be young again and says: 'I look upon retirement as the best period of life – I don't have to work for a living and so I can do as I like and I feel that now more than ever I can be creative in the way I use my time, and I can follow my desire to work with my community, to spend time with younger people and by doing this I feel my life's work can be passed on to the next generation, which is very satisfying. There are physical limitations to the amount of community work I can do, but then I am very happy to spend time writing – my goal now is to write the stories of my life.'

A spirit of anarchy, the refusal to sit down and be good, as much as anything inspire me and so I was delighted by a newspaper report of an old woman who stopped a street busker and asked: 'Were you playing?' The young man replied 'Yes', at which the woman told him: 'It were crap,' and ran off chortling fit to bust. Unkind perhaps but irresistibly spirited. Others may draw a certain hopefulness from the tale of Hilda Amiel remembered as a sweet, ever-chatty granny. Behind that façade was a mind quite definitely not dimmed by age: she masterminded the world's largest art counterfeiting scam worth £325 million, on the east coast of America.

I began this book distinctly gloomy about the fact that within what will probably seem little more than a spasm of time I shall be ending my mid-life decades, stepping off the bridge to join those who while I have been growing up have been so well disguised and diminished. But now I believe we can look forward with interest, alacrity and even enthusiasm.

In saying this I have drawn particular inspiration from the infinitely spirited, rigorous and engaging Baroness Barbara Castle, now eighty-four. I visited her at her home in the Chilterns with its view of bluebell woods and copper beeches. She sat in a deep chair, in the oak-beamed room, insisting I eat a biscuit while she told me about her own carefully planned diet, the morning exercises which were 'absolutely a must', the half-hour walk with the dog and then 'the mental stimulus of reading or writing something demanding enough that I know my mental faculties are still oiled'. Her autobiography which she said she had been determined to write before she died, had just been published. There are huge lunches, she described, given for the many nephews, nieces, partners and their children who compensate for the children she never had and help to offset the loneliness she still feels at the loss of her husband Ted. Our conversation – she hogged most of it – larky, hectoring, opinionated and utterly entertaining, ran over the time allotted and suddenly Baroness Castle realized she was weary and needed rest. But before I left she fixed me with a firm look and offered her simple adage on ageing successfully: 'You don't let old age happen to you – you happen to it.'

Bibliography

Too Long in the Tooth for Nirvana

Burroway, J. in J. Goldsworthy (ed.) *A Certain Age* (Virago Press 1993)

Coleman, P., Bond, J. and Peace, S. (eds.) *Ageing in Society* (Sage 1993)

Cowgill, D. *Ageing Around the World* (Wadsworth 1986)

De Beauvoir, S. *Old Age* (Andre Deutsch & Weidenfeld & Nicholson 1972)

Fisher, M. F. K. *Sister Age* (Chatto & Windus 1983)

Gerzon, M. *Coming into Our Own* (Delacorte Press 1993)

Hildebrand, P. *Beyond Mid-Life Crisis* (Sheldon Press 1995)

Jung, C. *Memories, Dreams and Reflections* (Fontana Press 1993)

Kupferman, J. *The MsTaken Body* (Robson Books 1979)

Lessing, D. *Summer Before the Dark* (Jonathan Cape 1973)

Meade, M. *Dorothy Parker, What Fresh Hell is This?* (Minerva 1991)

Sheehy, G. *Passages* (Bantam 1976)

Old, Moi?

Booth, W. *The Art of Growing Older* (Poseidon Press 1992)

Bull, R. and Ramsey, N. *The Social Psychology of Facial Appearance* (Springer Verlag 1988)

Coleman, P., Bond, J. and Peace, S. (eds.) *Ageing in Society* (Sage 1993)

Crowe, J. Ransom 'Piazza Piece', *The Penguin Book of Love Poetry* (Penguin 1973)

Davis, K. *Reshaping the Female Body* (Routledge 1994)

Freedman, R. *Beauty Bound* (Columbus Books 1986)

Gaer Luce, G. *Your Second Life* (Delacorte Press 1979)

Liggett, J. *The Human Face* (Constable 1974)

Lurie, A. *The Language of Clothes* (Random House NY 1981)

Milarepa, *The Hundred Thousand Songs of Milarepa*
(Shambala 1977)

Miles, R. *The Rites of Man* (Grafton Books 1991)

Moffat, M.J. (ed.) *Revelations: Diaries of Women* (Random
House 1975)

Paige, J. and Gordon, P. *Choice Years* (Ballantine Books
1991)

Parkin, M. in J. Goldsworthy (ed.) *A Certain Age* (Virago
Press 1993)

Waller, R. J. *The Bridges of Madison County* (Warner Books
Inc. 1992)

Wright, R. *The Moral Animal* (Pantheon Books NY 1994)

Critical Time

Friedan, B. *The Fountain of Age* (Jonathan Cape 1993)

Fry, A. *Safe Space* (Dent 1987)

Hesse, H. *Klingsor's Last Summer* (Picador 1952)

Heyn, D. *The Erotic Silence of the Married Woman*
(Bloomsbury 1992)

Hildebrand, P. *Beyond Mid-Life Crisis* (Sheldon Press 1995)

Kates Shulman, A. *Drinking the Rain* (Bloomsbury 1995)

Lawson, A. *Adultery* (Blackwell 1987)

Levinson, D. *The Seasons of a Man's Life* (Knopf NY 1978)

McCullin, D. *Unreasonable Behaviour* (Vintage 1990)

Matthew, C. *The Truth About Life After Forty, How to
Survive Middle Age* (Coronet 1983)

Pines, D. *A Woman's Unconscious Use of Her Body* (Virago
Press 1993)

Pinkola Estes, C. *Women Who Run With the Wolves*
(Rider 1992)

Reibstein, J. and Richards, M. *Sexual Arrangements* (Mandarin 1993)

Rutter, Michael & Marjorie, *Developing Minds* (Penguin 1992)

Seidler, V. *Men, Sex and Relationships* (Routledge 1992)

Look the Demon in the Eye

Apter, T. *Secret Paths* (W.W. Norton 1995)

Dychtwald, K. and Flower, J. *Agewave* (Bantam Books NY 1990)

Hildebrand, P. *Beyond Mid-Life Crisis* (Sheldon Press 1995)

Levinson, D. *The Seasons of a Man's Life* (Knopf NY 1978)

Luke, H. *Old Age* (Parabola Books NY 1987)

Mayer, N. *The Male Mid-Life Crisis* (Signet 1979)

Morrow Lindbergh, A. *A Gift From the Sea* (Chatto & Windus 1992)

Pines, D. *A Woman's Unconscious Use of Her Body* (Virago Press 1993)

Rowe, D. *Beyond Fear* (Fontana/Collins 1987)

Scott Peck, M. *The Road Less Travelled* (Arrow 1990)

Sheehy, G. *Passages* (Bantam 1976)

Weldon, F. *Female Friends* (Picador 1975)

Wilde McCormick, E. *Breakdown* (Optima 1993)

Yeats, W. B. 'The Second Coming', *The Collected Poems of W. B. Yeats* (Macmillan 1963)

Will You Still Need Me?

Banner, L. *In Full Flower* (Alfred A. Knopf 1992)

Bowskill, D. and Linacre, A. *The Male Menopause* (Goldsworthy, J. (ed.) Muller 1976)

Cauthery, P. and Stanway, A. & P., *The Complete Book of Love and Sex* (Century 1983)

Figes, E. in J. Goldsworthy (ed.) *A Certain Age* (Virago Press 1993)

Gibson, H. B. *The Emotional and Sexual Lives of Older People* (Chapman & Hall 1992)

Goldsworthy, J. (ed.) *A Certain Age* (Virago Press 1993)

Gomez, J. *Sixtysomething* (Thorsons 1993)

Greer, G. *The Change* (Penguin 1991)

Jukes, A. *Why Men Hate Women* (Free Association Books 1993)

Ojeda, L. *Menopause Without Medicine* (Thorsons 1990)

Reuben, D. *Everything You Wanted to Know About Sex, But Were Afraid to Ask* (Avon US 1979)

Vines, G. *Raging Hormones* (Virago Press 1993)

Wright, R. *The Moral Animal* (Pantheon NY 1994)

Living Like I Do

Porcino, J. *Living Longer, Living Better* (Crossroad US 1991)

Social Europe: A Survey for the European Year of Older People and Solidarity Between Generations (The Commission of the European Communities 1993)

Not Mellow But Outraged

Coleman, P., Bond, J. and Peace, S. (eds.) *Ageing in Society* (Sage 1993)

Handy C. *The Age of Unreason* (Business Books 1991), *The Empty Raincoat* (Hutchinson 1994)

Schuller, T. and Walker, A. *The Time of Our Life* (Institute of Public Policy Research 1990)

Looking Forward

Baker, J. *Tolstoy's Bicycle* (Panther Books 1985)

Castle, B. *Fighting all the Way* (Macmillan 1993)

Cosby, B. *Time Flies* (Bantam Books 1987)

Dytchwald, K. and Flower, J. *Agewave* (Bantam Books 1990)

Gomez, J. *Sixtysomething* (Thorsons 1993)

The Hen Co-op, *Growing Old Disgracefully* (Piatkus 1993)
Pullman, G. M. *The Art of Growing Older* (Poseidon Press
  1992)
Seidler, V. *Men, Sex and Relationships* (Routledge 1992)
Thompson, P., Itzin, C., and Abendstern M. *I Don't Feel Old*
  (Oxford University Press 1990)

Index

Index

children: dependence on, 261–2;
    empty-nest syndrome, 93, 108–19
Churchill, Winston, 183
Cicero, 214
Clarke, Maggie, 61–2
Cleveland, Pat, 66
clothes, 57–66
collagen injections, 42
Collagen UK, 273–4
Collins, Joan, 63
Coming of Age campaign, 291
Command Generation, 182, 352
Comme des Garçons, 66
Communique, 326
Community Care Act, 295
community living, 237–62
Compel, 278
Conran, Sir Terence, 225
Conservative Party, 295, 298
consultancies, 286–7
Cooke, Alistair, 310–11
Cooper, Professor Carey, 284–5
Cosby, Bill, 308, 345
counselling, 118, 165–7
Courcy, Anne de, 59
Cowgill, Donald, 18
La Crise, 82
Crosbie, Gilly, 292
Cruise, Tom, 39
Csikzentmihalyi, Mihaly, 149–50
Cunliffe, Lesley, 60

Daley, Janet, 334
Daniel, Jere, 309
Dante, 154
Dark Horse Venture, 333
Darker, Cec, 351
Darwall-Smith, Lucy, 263–5
Darwin, Charles, 190
Davidson, Max, 166
Davis, Kathy, 49, 55–6
death: awareness of, 8–9; in

communities, 256–7; denial of, 35,
    259–60; and mid-life crisis, 95
Delon, Alain, 68–9
demographic changes, 292–3
Deneuve, Catherine, 68, 189
denial, 145–8, 259–60
Denmark, 296, 297–8, 299
Dennis, Wayne, 347
dependence, 261–2
depression, 83, 85, 89, 113, 118–19
diet, 344, 346
Dietrich, Marlene, 189
discrimination *see* ageism
disposable income, 325–6
Donne, John, 178
Dubuffet, Mary, 338–9
Dychtwald, Ken, 162, 231–2, 284,
    287, 347
Dylan, Bob, 241

Eade, Anne, 263–5, 332
Eadie, Hannah, 333
Eager, Charlotte, 278
early retirement, 278–80, 284
Eastwood, Clint, 189
education, 313, 349–51
Eliot, T. S., 75, 94, 315
Ellis, Alice Thomas, 62, 68
Ellis, Havelock, 195
Ellison, Jeffrey, 284
Emerson, Ralph Waldo, 148–9
employment *see* work
empty-nest syndrome, 93, 108–19
Equal Opportunities Commission
    Institute of Personnel
    Development, 277
Erikson, Erik 89–90, 91, 92, 146
Ermisch, John, 294–5
Estes, Clarissa Pinkola, 106–7
Ethiopia, 18
Eurobarometer Survey, 272, 274,
    279, 294, 298, 300, 333

Index

Index